THE
VACCINE

THE
VACCINE

INSIDE THE RACE
TO CONQUER THE COVID-19 PANDEMIC

JOE MILLER with
DR. ÖZLEM TÜRECI and
DR. UĞUR ŞAHIN

ST. MARTIN'S
PRESS
NEW YORK

First published in the United States by St. Martin's Press,
an imprint of St. Martin's Publishing Group

THE VACCINE. Copyright © 2022 by Joe Miller, Uğur Şahin, and Özlem Türeci. All rights reserved. Printed in the United States of America. For information, address St. Martin's Publishing Group, 120 Broadway, New York, NY 10271.

www.stmartins.com

Designed by Steven Seighman

The Library of Congress Cataloging-in-Publication Data is available upon request.

ISBN 978-1-250-28036-7 (hardcover)
ISBN 978-1-250-28037-4 (ebook)

Our books may be purchased in bulk for promotional, educational, or business use. Please contact your local bookseller or the Macmillan Corporate and Premium Sales Department at 1-800-221-7945, extension 5442, or by email at MacmillanSpecialMarkets@macmillan.com.

First Edition: 2022

10 9 8 7 6 5 4 3 2 1

To my parents, thank you for staying safe

CONTENTS

Author's Note   ix

Prologue: The Coventry Miracle   1
1. The Outbreak   3
2. Project Lightspeed   30
3. The Unknowns   61
4. The mRNA Biohackers   82
5. The Tests   108
6. Forging Alliances   128
7. First in Human   158
8. On Our Own   179
9. It Works!   211
10. The New Normal   230
     Epilogue   246

     Appendix   249
     Acknowledgments   251
     Notes   253
     Index   271

AUTHOR'S NOTE

Writing a book about a pandemic, during a pandemic, was a surreal experience. I was able to meet just a handful of the sixty people I interviewed, for a combined total of over one hundred fifty hours, in person. I could only travel to two locations—Mainz and Marburg.

Consequently, sketches of characters and places occasionally rely on descriptions provided by others. Understandably, memories of a taxing year proved sometimes to be imperfect, and the dates and times provided by witnesses to the same events were contradictory. Wherever possible, I have independently verified the facts, but some events in the book are based on the best recollections of one or two observers. Similarly, quoted speech represents an approximation of what was actually said, built on the reports of those involved, and, when feasible, sense-checked with others who were in the (often virtual) room.

Some place-names and identifying features have been changed or omitted at the request of security services charged with protecting BioNTech and its suppliers from ongoing threats. Other parts of the supply chain have not been defined in detail, for similar reasons. None of these choices undermine the integrity of the story.

There were a thousand ways to tell this tale, and I had to choose one, in the time allowed. This is the first draft of history.

—Joe Miller

PROLOGUE: THE COVENTRY MIRACLE

It was the shot *seen* around the world.

On a frigid December morning, soon after the clock struck half past six in the outpatient ward of the UK's University Hospital, Coventry, ninety-year-old Maggie Keenan lowered her spotted gray cardigan, rolled up a blue MERRY CHRISTMAS T-shirt, and averted her gaze while a nurse[1] emptied the contents of a syringe into her left arm. Under the glare of a dozen TV lights, the retired jewelry shop assistant, pearly eyes sparkling above a blue disposable mask, became the first patient on earth to receive a fully tested and approved vaccine against a virus that had already claimed the lives of 1.5 million people. For eleven months, humankind had been almost as defenseless against COVID-19 as it had been when the so-called Spanish flu killed tens of millions, including thousands in Coventry, over a century ago. Now, science was fighting back. In the hospital's parking lot, reporters adjusted their earpieces, looked down camera lenses, and brought the news to weary viewers across the globe: *help was on its way.*

Recuperating inside the hospital with a cup of tea, Maggie, who was to turn ninety-one the following week, told reporters the jab was "the best early birthday present" and talked of how she was looking forward to finally hugging her four grandchildren after months in self-isolation.[2] Before she was wheeled out of the ward under a guard of honor formed by doctors and nurses, the vial and syringe used for her historic injection were whisked off to the Science Museum in London. There, they would be permanently displayed alongside a lancet once owned by Edward Jenner,[3] who paved the way for modern vaccinations in 1796 by inoculating his gardener's son against smallpox in an English town just seventy miles from where Maggie had received her lifesaving drug. The exhibit, curators hoped, would forever tell the tale of how, in humankind's darkest hour for a generation, COVID-19 was quashed by the timely arrival of a medical marvel.

What the small ampoule will not convey, however, is just how unlikely its existence was at the end of 2020. Although vaccine technology had come a long way since Jenner's experiments, the process of creating and testing a new drug remained fraught with risk. A study of thousands of clinical trials that had taken place in the twenty years prior to the discovery of the novel coronavirus found that even when backed with billions of dollars of funding from the world's largest pharmaceutical companies, roughly 60 percent of all vaccine projects failed.[4] In February 2020, Anthony Fauci, America's leading infectious diseases expert, had warned that even though pharmaceutical companies and regulators were working on accelerating the drug development process to respond to an emergency, a vaccine was a year away "at best."[5] The World Health Organization's chief, Tedros Adhanom Ghebreyesus, predicted that it would take eighteen months for a viable jab to emerge, never mind be authorized for public use.

Nine months later, an extraordinarily effective vaccine, based on a platform that had never before been used in a licensed pharmaceutical, would be available thanks to the efforts of two previously sidelined scientists in the German city of Mainz. For decades, the husband-and-wife team had believed that a tiny molecule shunned by the pharmaceutical establishment could herald a revolution in medicine by harnessing the powers of the immune system.

They did not think it would take a deadly pandemic to prove them right.

1

THE OUTBREAK

For the first time in weeks, Uğur Şahin's calendar was clear. It was a Friday morning and the two-bedroom apartment he shared with his wife, Özlem Türeci, and their teenage daughter was unusually empty. In the silence, he scrolled through his Spotify library and settled on a well-worn playlist. As he sat at his computer, cradling a steaming-hot cup of oolong tea, the Turkish-born immunologist's makeshift office filled with the soothing sounds of recorded birdsong.

Uğur's inbox was overflowing, and he had barely begun to look through submissions from his Ph.D. students when Özlem and their daughter, back from work and school, popped their heads around the door to remind him that it was 4:00 p.m.: time for phở and banh mi at their favorite Vietnamese restaurant. The family rarely skipped this weekly ritual, especially if one of them had recently been away. It was the early evening before they all returned home and Uğur could return to his desk to indulge his only real hobby—catching up on reading.

A constantly active mind, this was the professor's idea of relaxation. Disdain for time-wasting was one of the many traits Uğur shared with Özlem, whom he'd met almost thirty years earlier on rotation at a cancer ward. He was a young physician; she was in her final year at med school. The couple, now partners in science, business, and life, had never owned a TV and stayed off social media, relying instead on select online publications they considered worthy of their attention. Uğur's home workstation, consisting of two large screens that would not look out of place on an investment bank's trading floor, was their portal to the rest of the world.

Opening his internet browser, Uğur started methodically making his way through a list of bookmarked websites. It was January 24, and the year 2020 had started slowly in Germany. Local media outlets in his adopted city of Mainz were covering an environmental protest in which schoolkids had blocked traffic for miles. *Der Spiegel,* one of Germany's most respected magazines, led its home page with a story on the rise, and questionable ethics, of German gangster rap. Inside the week's digital issue were articles speculating whether infighting in the Democratic Party would effectively hand Donald Trump reelection in the United States and an analysis of the cyberwar being waged by the kingdom of Saudi Arabia, which stood accused of hacking Amazon founder Jeff Bezos's phone. Tucked away in the science section was a report from the Chinese megacity of Wuhan, which had been beset by a novel respiratory illness.

The fifty or so cases of this illness monitored by local authorities seemed to have been traced back to the Huanan wholesale "wet market," which sold seafood, live poultry, bats, snakes, and marmots, some of which were slaughtered on-site. Although it was too early to draw any conclusions, the evidence pointed to a development that sent shivers down the spines of epidemiologists—so-called cross-species transmission. In other words, a virus had probably passed from animals to people, catching humans completely off guard. An evolutionary arms race was underway between this frightening new foe and the combined forces of the human immune system.

The piece piqued Uğur's interest somewhat, as he had devoted his adult life to understanding how the immune system marshals its disparate troops to fight disease. The company he had founded with Özlem eleven years earlier, BioNTech, had embarked on projects to develop flu, HIV, and tuberculosis vaccines. But pesky viruses were only of mild concern to the fifty-four-year-old. Only a dozen or so of Uğur's thousand-plus staff were developing drugs to fight communicable infections. The rest were focused on the couple's core mission: curing cancer. At long last, they were on the brink of a breakthrough.

It was this message—that a cure for some cancers may be in reach—that Uğur had taken to a familiar stage nineteen days earlier, in San Francisco. For more than a decade, his working year would kick off in one of the windowless ballrooms of the city's Westin St. Francis hotel, where he would painstakingly present his plan to develop next-generation cancer treatments at the biotechnology industry's most important showcase, the J. P. Morgan Health Care Conference.

This event had turned into an annual pilgrimage for the pharma world, a corporate circus that attracted tens of thousands of scientists, entrepreneurs, and investors. Hundreds of start-ups shelled out more than $1,000 a night[1] for downtown hotel rooms in the hopes of pitching their wares to deep-pocketed fund managers. Uğur, a softly spoken teetotaler who hated hyperbole and was almost allergic to the networking that formed a key part of the four-day symposium, was hardly the center of attention. The media hype at the dealmaking event was focused on Silicon Valley darlings, those who claimed to have a formula for exponential growth. BioNTech's data-driven talks were usually delivered to an audience consisting of a few dozen mid-ranking executives and venture capitalists, some of whom wore an expression that suggested they may have absent-mindedly wandered into the wrong hall.

This January, however, the reception had been different. When Uğur made his way to the dais—having swapped his usual uniform of plain-colored tees for a collared shirt and suit jacket—almost two hundred people turned their attention to the projector screen above his buzz-cut head.

His presentation had been uploaded onto the internet—as required by market regulators—with only moments to spare, thanks to Uğur's unusual routines. He hated losing days to jet lag and tried to stay on German time while on short trips. After the sixteen-hour journey from Mainz to California, he had gone straight to sleep without finalizing his slides and woken up at 2:00 a.m. on the day of the big speech to work on them instead. Uğur had a tough time condensing all that he wanted to

communicate into a twenty-minute talk, and when his colleagues surfaced hours later, they found their boss surrounded by coffee and the
remains of Starbucks brownies he had brought with him from home,
still making the final touches to his precious PowerPoint.

Uğur needn't have been so concerned. Shares in BioNTech were on
a tear and had more than tripled in the three months since their disappointing debut on New York's Nasdaq stock exchange, which had taken
place during an economic downturn. The company was on the cusp of
launching seven clinical trials for drugs that would tackle solid tumors
such as advanced melanoma. Onstage, Uğur ran through these achievements in detail, fighting the urge to delve more deeply into the science,
about which he was far more passionate than commercial milestones. The
audience, composed largely of specialists in the sector, seemed enthralled.
That year, 2020, Uğur told the crowd, would be the year BioNTech proved
the doubters wrong.

There was no time to lose. Soon after he'd finished his talk, Uğur
hopped on a plane to Seattle, where he met with a team at the Bill &
Melinda Gates Foundation, which had recently signed a $100 million
agreement with BioNTech to develop a slew of new drugs. Hours later, he
moved on to Boston, to stop by a small cancer immunotherapy company
that BioNTech was about to purchase in a $67 million deal. The purpose
of the visit was to reassure staff that he, a fellow scientist, was interested in
advancing their innovations and was not a vulture disguised in a lab coat
who had come to gut the firm and slim down its workforce. At this point,
Uğur was still fairly oblivious to events in Wuhan. He walked around the
biotech firm's foyer, introducing himself to dozens of soon-to-be employees, shaking each of them vigorously by the hand.

As he jetted from airport to airport, country to country, Uğur heard
further mention of the outbreak in China and engaged in a few casual
conversations with friends and colleagues about the new disease. But the
topic hadn't really aroused his curiosity. Pathogens that broke the species
barrier, known as *zoonotic viruses,* weren't uncommon, and the likelihood of a small cluster of infections leading to a public health crisis was

minimal. Uğur, a busy man facing a very busy fortnight, didn't think much of it.

That is, until that Friday evening back in Mainz, stomach sated by phở and his calendar as clear as it ever got. Scrolling through carefully saved tabs, Uğur's attention drifted to his favorite material: prominent academic journals such as *Nature* and *Science*—which often featured contributions from the team he ran with Özlem—and to the home page of *The Lancet,* one of the world's oldest and most respected medical publications. There, his eye settled on a submission from more than twenty Hong Kong–based researchers, which offered an analysis of a "familial cluster of pneumonia associated with the 2019 novel coronavirus." It was the second part of the title that led Uğur to click: "indicating person-to-person transmission."

The ten-page study succinctly analyzed how a new disease had spread among five members of a family who had recently returned to their home in China's tech capital, Shenzhen, after a weeklong trip to Wuhan. The authors had become aware of the cases when the quintet checked in to an enormous teaching hospital run by the University of Hong Kong, with symptoms including fever, diarrhea, and severe coughing. Intrigued, doctors ran a series of lung x-rays, gathered blood, urine, and fecal samples from their subjects, and tested them for evidence of everything from the common cold to influenza to bacterial infections like chlamydia. But the results all came back negative.

Flummoxed, the researchers took nasal swabs and saliva samples from the infected family to extract and analyze the genetic sequence of this mysterious malady. They found it to be closely related to several coronaviruses, particularly a subset that scientists had thought was confined to bats. This pathogen bore all the hallmarks of the novel disease recently discovered in Wuhan. But when questioned, the five insisted that they had never been anywhere near the city's wet markets during their visit, nor had they handled any animals, alive or dead. They had not sampled game meat delicacies in local restaurants; in fact, they had relied on the home cooking of their three aunts in the city throughout their stay.

Two members of the family—the mother and daughter—had, however, visited relatives who were being treated for febrile pneumonia in a Wuhan hospital. They fell ill soon after. As did the father, son-in-law, and grandson. Strikingly, when the five returned to their home in Shenzhen, another relative—who had not been on the trip—started suffering from back pain and felt weak, before developing a fever and dry cough and being admitted to the hospital.

This last revelation startled Uğur. He slid his chair back from the desk, stared out of the window at the distant spires of Mainz's thousand-year-old cathedral, and began to process the implications of this information. It suggested to him that contact with animals was merely the source of the disease, which, now that it was unleashed in humans, was spreading like wildfire from person to person and infecting the broader population in cities across China. That alone was cause for significant alarm, but there was another detail in the paper that Uğur found even more terrifying. A sixth family member had been on the trip to Wuhan—the seven-year-old granddaughter. She felt completely fine, but doctors in Shenzhen tested her anyhow and found her to be positive for the new coronavirus. This suggested that, unlike the SARS-CoV outbreak of 2002,[2] here was a pathogen that could travel undetected between perfectly healthy people. It was, in effect, a silent assassin.

Uğur's mind started racing. He was no infectious disease expert, but he'd lived through the SARS-CoV outbreak and its successor that emerged in Saudi Arabia a decade later, known as the Middle East respiratory syndrome, or MERS, and out of curiosity, he had studied the data modeling that had predicted their rapid spread. If this new virus could circulate incognito, making it impossible for health authorities to identify who might be contagious, it would become uncontrollable within days. The dark, but logical effect, Uğur suddenly realized, was that all human contact would be considered perilous, ripping apart families, societies, and the global economy. This extreme revelation, which would have been dismissed out of hand by any casual observer at the time, proved to be remarkably prescient within just a few months.

The central question was, how much damage had already been done? The study's authors seemed convinced that they were witnessing "an early stage of the epidemic" and urged authorities "to isolate patients and trace and quarantine contacts as early as possible." Instinctively, Uğur felt they were underplaying the threat. But he needed more data. Having barely heard of Wuhan before reading the paper, he had half assumed that it must be a small city. The fact that it was often described as being in Hubei Province made the metropolis sound somewhat provincial too. A quick Google search set him straight. Wuhan had at least eleven million citizens, making it more populous than London, New York, or Paris. A YouTube video showed off its modern and extensive metro underground system. Next, he looked up plane and train connections from the city. Were he a man in the habit of using profanity, his findings would have made him swear profusely. There were 2,300 scheduled flights a week, to and from locations across China, as well as global hubs like New York, London, and Tokyo. Its rail timetables were almost all in Mandarin and harder to decipher, but it was clear that Wuhan was home to three major interchanges with regular links to the entire region. To make matters worse, Uğur discovered that it was currently the Chunyun, or spring festival season, during which workers who had moved to China's megacities traveled back home to visit friends and family in rural areas. Roughly three billion trips would be made during the period, in one of the largest human migrations on the planet.

What was unfolding, Uğur realized, was a nightmare scenario, one he had heard described by colleagues who monitored such matters. Globalization had long been making life a lot easier for infectious diseases, which for centuries could only spread as fast and as far as people could walk, horses could gallop, or ships could sail.[3] Outbreaks were now more common and were turning into epidemics with alarming frequency. The emergence of a new pathogen that could be spread unwittingly by healthy people in one of the most connected and populous cities on earth provided an almost perfect platform for a pandemic.

Initial local containment measures, such as preventing those with a fever from traveling on public transport, were woefully insufficient. Uğur could not find reliable statistics on how much global travel had increased since the outbreak of SARS-CoV, but he estimated that ten times as many passengers were hopping to and from China, as well as within the country, compared to 2003. Assuming the whole human population was susceptible to this new coronavirus, Uğur estimated a transmission rate of between 2 and 7, meaning that each person carrying the disease would spread it to at least a couple of others, and possibly several more. Even with the limited available data on deaths from the new disease, he worked out that the mortality rate would be somewhere between 0.3 to 10, out of every 100 people infected, with the elderly on the higher end of that macabre scale. In the *best*-case scenario, that would mean 2 million deaths worldwide, far surpassing recent epidemics.

By this measure, Uğur and his family could soon be in as much danger as residents in Wuhan. But his reflexes were rigidly scientific. As a practicing doctor, he had exposed himself to disease in the past and was not a hypochondriac. His interest was in the arithmetic. Uğur told a friend soon afterward, "I understood instantly that we were going to face two potential scenarios: either a very fast pandemic which kills millions within a couple of months, or a prolonged epidemic situation which will last for the next sixteen to eighteen months." To give scientists a fighting chance, he hoped it "would be the latter."

Stepping away from his computer once again, Uğur wondered if he had let his imagination run away with him. Even in a world with relatively cheap and regular long-distance travel, major pandemics were rare. The last two novel coronaviruses—causing SARS and MERS—had sent headline writers and health organizations into a frenzy. While controlling their spread had not been a trivial matter, the epidemics petered out almost as quickly as they had appeared, after some localized lockdowns and mandatory mask-wearing. But while he was no epidemiologist, Uğur was a keen mathematician. In the late 1980s, he had even squeezed in a mathematics correspondence course, while studying medicine, and maintained an interest in the subject. "He read complex maths books like others read novels," says Helma Heinen, who served as the couple's assistant for two decades. The situation Uğur was learning about in January 2020 lent itself to relatively simple computation. All the ingredients were there for something serious: a known virus class that had already produced two deadly outbreaks—SARS had killed more than 770,[4] MERS more than

850[5]—no preexisting immunity in the majority of the population, fast and asymptomatic human-to-human transmission, and infected patients probably already sitting on planes jetting all over the world.

While he was reading, real-world validation of his hypothesis was provided by French health authorities, who announced that three people, recently arrived from China and hospitalized in Paris and Bordeaux, had tested positive for the novel coronavirus, making them the first confirmed cases in Europe. Even closer to home, Mainz's university hospital, at which Uğur and Özlem both taught, announced that it had established procedures for dealing with coronavirus patients,[6] due to its proximity to Frankfurt Airport, which was still welcoming 190,000 passengers each day.[7]

Tentatively, Uğur typed out an email to BioNTech's chairman, Helmut Jeggle, who managed the affairs of the company's billionaire backers. The two would chat regularly on weekends, and a call was scheduled for the very next day. After its lackluster IPO, the company's coffers were not overflowing, and Uğur knew he needed to prepare the ground for dealing with this threat. "There is a new type of virus around, which is passed from person to person," he wrote. "It is highly unpredictable." He thought about adding more detail on his findings but, knowing Helmut, decided it was better to wait until they were speaking on the phone. As midnight drew near, Uğur clicked Send.

The next morning, after a restless night's sleep, Uğur entered the kitchen to find Özlem and their daughter preparing breakfast, having returned from the local farmers' market with a haul of fresh bread and eggs. As he lent a hand, frying vegetables and making omelets, Uğur began bombarding his family with his findings. This was by no means unusual—Friday, Saturday, and Sunday were "science days" in their household ("We never talk about anything else, actually," their daughter jokes), during which the couple, undisturbed by meetings and emails, tried to focus on catching up with and discussing the latest research in their fields.

Nor was there anything surprising about the boldness of Uğur's prognosis; that the world was already in the midst of a pandemic, but just didn't know it yet. Even during their first dates in the early 1990s, the young doctor would quote verbatim from new scientific publications, drawing grand conclusions about innovations that would shape the future of medicine. Özlem—a doctor and scientist in her own right—had initially found Uğur's tendency to issue such predictions annoying. But in the years that followed, during which the duo authored hundreds of academic papers, filed hundreds of patents, founded two nonprofit organizations, and established two billion-euro businesses in the face of skepticism from much of the medical establishment, they had developed a deep respect for each other's instincts. "He has a very high hit rate when it comes to predicting outcomes based on complex data or complicated situations," says Özlem, "so I took him very seriously."

In his deliberate, detailed manner, Uğur outlined what would happen next. The virus, he said, would spread in densely populated areas at such speed that lockdowns would be inevitable. "We will most likely see schools closed by April," he told the family. At the time, with a total of five cases confirmed outside of Asia, including just two in the USA, that seemed like a ridiculous assertion. "Experts with a deep understanding of previous outbreaks seemed fairly confident that this one would come and go," Uğur recalls. "But I said to Özlem, 'This time, it is different.'" Soon, he believed, humanity would be left to tackle this virus with nothing but the rudimentary tools used to contain pandemics in the eighteenth-century: quarantines, social distancing, basic hygiene measures, and restrictions on movement.

Unless, of course, there was a vaccine.

When it came to his phone call with Helmut later that day, Uğur knew he still had some convincing to do. The company was not flush with cash—in fact, there was just over €600 million left in the kitty (not a large sum in biotech terms)—and BioNTech was already thinking carefully about allocating its limited resources in what was going to be a busy year. But ever since they had shaken hands at a retreat near Frankfurt, twelve years earlier, when Helmut's bosses agreed to invest €150 million into founding

BioNTech, the two had developed a rare bond. Impressed by the precision of Uğur and Özlem's science, Helmut rarely dismissed their outlandish ideas out of hand. Just a year earlier, soon after the J. P. Morgan conference, Uğur had convinced Helmut that BioNTech should buy a small, specialist antibody company in San Diego that had just filed for bankruptcy, even though its products bore little relation to those being developed in Mainz. This ask, Uğur knew, was orders of magnitude bigger, so he started with a tentative suggestion: "I think we can create something to fight this."

Helmut, an economist by training, was surprised that Uğur was taking the new virus so seriously. Since receiving Uğur's email the night before, he had done some basic research on the Wuhan outbreak and could detect little alarm among governments beyond Chinese shores. But Uğur was unequivocal: this outbreak had the potential to be as bad as the Asian flu pandemic that had rocked the world in the late 1950s. "It is more than a premonition," Uğur insisted. His expertise, when distilled to its essence, was in identifying patterns and connecting dots. "A pattern," he said in a definitive tone, "never lies." Helmut hung up and immediately searched for the Asian flu pandemic on Wikipedia. He was astonished by the death count: up to four million. Convinced there had been some mistake, he messaged Uğur, asking if he was really predicting such a calamity, despite the enormous advances in medicine and health care made in the intervening decades. "Yes," Uğur replied within minutes, "it could even be worse."

Unbeknownst to Helmut, Uğur had already taken action. Before sitting down to watch a Marvel movie with the family—another weekly ritual—he had sent a few BioNTech specialists the genetic sequence of this new virus and told them to prepare for detailed discussions first thing Monday morning.

Looking back, as I write this in the summer of 2021, the fact that the novel coronavirus could be controlled by a vaccine is almost taken for granted. But sitting on the sofas in their cluttered living room on that Saturday evening, surrounded by floor-to-ceiling bookshelves, Uğur and Özlem knew that anyone attempting to design an effective jab would need much more than mere scientific excellence to be successful. They would also need an extraordinary amount of good fortune.

For a start, there was never a guarantee that *any* new virus could be targeted by a vaccine. Attempts at producing a prophylactic for HIV/AIDS, for example, had not only failed but in some cases exacerbated the disease. Second, virtually nothing was known about this new coronavirus. No one had much of a clue which parts of the complex human immune system were needed to combat natural infection, or whether those who recovered from the disease it caused would develop long-lasting immunity. There had been no successful vaccine developed against closely related coronaviruses that could help Uğur and Özlem gauge the probability of victory against the one discovered in Wuhan. Scientists had scrambled to develop vaccines in response to the previous outbreaks of SARS and MERS, but the two diseases faded from view before a vaccine could be clinically tested. There was no blueprint, no road map, no set of instructions for battling this pathogen.

Uğur and Özlem also knew that previous attempts at designing vaccines from scratch—and getting them approved for emergency use—had taken an age. In 1967, American microbiologist Maurice Hilleman set the modern record, by delivering a licensed mumps jab less than five years after he realized his daughter had caught the disease. More recently, the development of a vaccine for Ebola had taken five years too, and that was with the might of the world's largest and most experienced vaccine-maker, Merck, behind the project, as well as hundreds of millions of dollars of investment and a fast-tracked regulatory process.

Even tweaking well-established pharmaceuticals was a slow process. During the 2009 swine flu outbreak, at the behest of the Obama administration, manufacturers had quickly modified influenza vaccines—using a decades-old method involving fertilized chicken eggs. They received emergency approval in six months, but this still meant that they missed the second wave in the USA. Only thirty million doses were available in the U.S. by the end of October,[8] and that was despite scientists addressing a virus family that was well studied by vaccinologists and leveraging a vaccine technology that was in widespread use. The outbreak led to an estimated 12,500 deaths. The vaccine, the Centers for Disease Control and Prevention later calculated, only managed to save 300 lives.[9]

Unlike the pharma giants that developed those vaccines, Uğur and Özlem had an ace up their sleeve, one on which they had staked their professional reputations. With it, as Uğur had sketched out in San Francisco, they hoped to revolutionize the way cancers were treated. If exploited correctly, they believed, it could even stop infectious disease outbreaks and do so in record time. Their trump card was a microscopic, unloved molecule, known as mRNA.

The couple's first encounter with this form of RNA, which stands for *ribonucleic acid,* was almost as fortuitous as their own meeting. Uğur and Özlem were both born in the 1960s to Turkish parents who'd made their way to West Germany after the government signed an immigration agreement with Ankara to boost its dilapidated postwar labor force. They grew up within 150 miles of each other and pursued remarkably similar paths that would eventually converge in a fairy-tale manner.

While his father worked at the Ford car factory in Cologne, Uğur, the oldest of two children, was devouring popular-science documentaries on TV, presented by the German equivalent of Neil deGrasse Tyson, Hoimar von Ditfurth. "All nerd kids watched him," says Özlem, including herself. Uğur also read English magazines like *Scientific American* and, from the age of eleven, was struck by the beauty and complexity of the immune system. He was desperate to learn more about it, but that was no easy task. "We didn't have Google," Uğur points out, "so every time my mother and I went into town, I headed to the bookstore." The young Uğur also had a good relationship with a friendly local librarian, who ordered new science and math books for him and set them aside for when he came in.

"I also always wanted to become a doctor," Uğur says. An aunt in Turkey, he remembers, was suffering from breast cancer, and he was puzzled by the disease. "Even as a child, I couldn't get it into my head that people with cancer look healthy, but are terminally ill." Adults seemed resigned to this reality, but Uğur felt a sense of urgency. Something, surely, could be done.

Three hours' drive to the north of Cologne, Özlem's father, a surgeon who had a keen interest in technology and science, was playing a more direct role in his offspring's early medical education. He had come to Germany two years before her birth to avoid being sent by his government to serve as a doctor in the majority Kurdish region of Turkey, where sectarian tensions were simmering. Since he had not trained in the country, it was down to the whim of Germany's Ärztekammern, or medical councils, to decide on his placement. As a result, Özlem's family ended up in Lastrup, a small town in Lower Saxony surrounded by farms, where her father became the sole doctor in the local hospital. A converted Catholic convent, this institution was staffed exclusively by nuns. "My dad was the only man, the only physician, Turkish, and Muslim," Özlem remembers.

Alone in a rural region, Özlem's father quickly became a master of all medical disciplines, a de facto general practitioner, seeing to the wounds of locals gored by bulls, and even occasionally acting as a vet, while also performing invasive procedures. From a young age, Özlem would follow her father as he did his rounds—the hospital was across the street from their home—even into the operating theater. The eldest of two girls, she had watched her first appendectomy at the age of six. This gory exposure did not dent her enthusiasm for the profession, and as she grew older, her ambition was to do similar work as the nuns. She watched as they performed all the roles assumed these days by hospital staff, nurses, and junior doctors—from cooking meals for patients, to wrapping arms in casts, to assisting in surgery—and longed to play a part.

In a society that still treated immigrants, especially those of a different ethnicity, with some suspicion, Uğur and Özlem excelled at school. "It was very important for my parents that I study," says Uğur. "They worked every day, they woke up at 4:30 in the morning and then went to work because they had the dream that their children could become something better."[10] That dream went some way to being fulfilled when, in 1984, Uğur finished at the top of his class at what is now called the Erich Kästner Gymnasium in Cologne, becoming the first child of a so-called guest worker to complete an Abitur—the German version of A-levels or SATs—in its eighteen-year history. Özlem, whose teenage years were split between schools in the spa towns of Bad Driburg and later Bad Harzburg—both of which are home to fewer than twenty thousand people—was educated in a similarly homogenous environment, where she was the only child of migrants among her peers. There was not even much of a Turkish community in the broader region—most of her father's compatriots had headed to Germany's centers of heavy industry, such as the Ruhr valley. An introverted but diligent student, Özlem busied herself with extracurricular activities, including, naturally, the science club.

Although he was a handy footballer—a self-described "relentless midfielder"—there was little doubt as to what Uğur's future had in store for him. At his graduation party, one classmate remembers a discussion among a group who had taken up cigarettes, in which someone joked: "Why should we stop smoking? Uğur is going into medicine anyway."[11] But even as a teenager, Uğur knew he wanted to combine research with real-life experience. At Cologne's university, which traced its roots to the Holy Roman Empire, Uğur trod that very academic path, combining a medical degree with a doctorate in immunotherapy.

Two years later, when Özlem graduated from high school, she took an almost identical route at the Saarland University, in Germany's smallest state, studying for an MD while simultaneously doing lab work for a Ph.D. in molecular biology.

By chance, Uğur soon ended up in Saarland too, where he did a placement at the university hospital in Homburg, a small town just twenty miles from the French border. In 1991, amid frenzied commutes between lectures, hospital wards, and research labs, the two met in what Özlem describes as "a scene out of a movie," although it was far from the most romantic of settings. She was on rotation at a blood cancer ward, where Uğur was a junior resident and her supervisor/mentor. Most of the patients were in the last-chance saloon, and the pair often found themselves having to tell those under their care that all available therapeutic options had been exhausted. Every single day, they watched people succumb to this unforgiving illness, often without so much as a friendly hand to squeeze in their final moments. It was amid this horror, while doing the afternoon rounds, that they caught each other's eye.

The young lovers soon found out that they had much more in common than similar backgrounds. Both were frustrated by the limited tools they had at their disposal to treat long-suffering patients. Physicians could only choose between the blunt instruments of surgery, chemotherapy and radiation, crudely referred to in their profession as "cut, poison, burn." Meanwhile, in the lab, Uğur and Özlem caught a glimpse of the cutting-edge technologies that could revolutionize cancer medicine. The disparity between scientific theory and clinical practice in this life-or-death field gnawed at them. Not content with treating the symptoms of the disease, they longed to be involved in its prevention and in finding cures. This bench-to-bedside approach, which aimed to bring new drugs to patients as soon as possible, would, years later, be dubbed "translational medicine." With it, an entirely new discipline would emerge. But back then, in the early 1990s, the pair would not have been able to define it in such grand terms. All they knew was that they wanted to do science, but not for science's sake. At heart, Uğur was still the boy shocked at adults' blithe acceptance of a terminal diagnosis. Özlem was still the girl who longed to emulate her father, the all-around healer. They committed to each other and to working together to beat back the cruel disease consuming those around them.

Famously dubbed the "emperor of all maladies" by oncologist Siddhartha Mukherjee, cancer presented a unique challenge. Unlike viruses or bacteria, which invade the body after coming to life elsewhere, carcinogenic cells are produced at breakneck speed by healthy cells that randomly acquire mutations over time and, at some point, start to grow in an uncontrolled manner. They are designed to cause maximum harm to their hosts. As such, they are essentially a traitor within the ranks, a foe wearing the uniform of a friend, which the immune system fails to perceive as a threat.

For more than two centuries, scientists had understood that the body could be trained to detect an external enemy, such as an infectious disease, and instructed to tool up for any future encounters with a similar assailant. It was this observation that led to the development of vaccines that have saved hundreds of millions of lives. What a small community of immunologists worldwide were beginning to understand in the early 1990s was that the immune system could also be trained to recognize and fight *internal* threats and that this would pave the way for a new class of cancer medicine. But immunotherapy, as this nascent field was called, was at this time confined largely to university campuses, far off the radar of the pharmaceutical industry.

Uğur and Özlem were members of this niche club. The patients perishing on their watch, they believed, already had weapons coursing through their veins to fight tumors. They just had to find a way of harnessing these powers and of unleashing them against this sophisticated disease.

The immune system is an army with highly organized, highly specialized units. Each of these units receives its orders in a different way, wears a different uniform, and employs a distinctive combat technique. But once an enemy is clearly identified, the separate units are mobilized in unison to perform a massive, multipronged, and coordinated counterattack.

When on song, the beauty of the immune system is that it combines precision with potency. Weapons such as antibodies and T-cells, the sharpshooters of the immune army, attack with great force once they recognize a specific molecule as their target. What scientists were beginning to discover, as Uğur and Özlem turned their attention to cancer, was that tumors are dotted with distinctive molecules not found on healthy cells. If the immune system could be taught to recognize them, the snipers could get cancer cells in their sights and open fire.

After Özlem abandoned her medical training in 1994 to dedicate herself to research, the pair, whose preoccupation she describes with a wry smile as "immune system whisperers," spent years on the hunt for those distinctive molecules—known as *antigens*. Their aim was to reproduce them in a lab setting and introduce antigens into patients, where they would function like a wanted poster; a clear instruction to apprehend and attack anything that resembled the enemy. The body would hopefully take a good, hard look at this felon, generate a comprehensive immune response, and, recognizing the antigen's resemblance to those of tumors, treat those cells as enemies too.

In principle, there were several ways to introduce an antigen into the body, and the couple tried them all. "We were typical nerds," Özlem, who, on occasion, proudly wears a T-shirt with an illustrated version of the Schrödinger's cat paradox, readily admits. "We were broadly interested in lots of different technologies, and none of them were accepted." But they found that methods such as synthetic peptides, recombinant proteins, DNA, or viral vectors (later to be used by Oxford and Astra-Zeneca for their COVID-19 jab) came with limitations. Either they required cell cultures to be grown in a petri dish—a tricky and lengthy process—or they were not able to prompt a strong and sustainable immune response.

Then, in the mid-1990s, Uğur and Özlem came across the most niche platform of them all, the trump card that they would play decades later to develop a coronavirus vaccine. It was based on RNA.

Believed by some to be the original biomolecule from which the rest of life evolved, RNA has an extraordinary set of abilities. First discovered in the late nineteenth century, it can, like its more celebrated cousin DNA, store genetic information. But RNA also acts as what scientists call a *catalyst*, meaning it can make copies of itself[12] without the help of other molecules. At the dawn of time, the theory goes, an RNA molecule carried a cellular blueprint *and* created the chemical reactions necessary to build something with it. It was both the first chicken and the first egg.

Uğur and Özlem, however, were interested in a far more prosaic function of RNA, which was first sketched by a group of academics huddled over a side table in the middle of a raucous party at the start of the Swinging Sixties[13] in Cambridge, UK. They had discovered that a version of the molecule, which exists in the cells of every human being and animal, was essentially the biological equivalent of a courier with a code. It carried a set of instructions from the DNA of a cell to the "factory" part of the cell, where the code was used to create the essential proteins that build and control the body's organs and tissues. Once this mission was complete, the single-stranded, ribbonlike structure was destroyed, often within minutes. In the autumn of 1960, it was given a name: messenger RNA. Soon shortened to mRNA, the molecule remained an object of fascination for those interested in gaining a better understanding of the natural world, but was largely ignored by clinical researchers. No one won a Nobel Prize for mRNA discoveries, and Big Pharma hardly gave it a second glance. Mention of mRNA-based drugs at scientific conferences was either ignored or met with ridicule—and not entirely without justification.

First, the molecule was notoriously unstable in a laboratory setting. Naked RNA, outside of cells, would degrade within seconds, thanks to ubiquitous enzymes in the air and on surfaces, that have a kryptonite-like effect on the tiny organism. A single cough, for example, could kill it dead. Even if kept alive in a so-called clean room, no one had managed to work out how to stop mRNA from being instantly disintegrated once introduced into the body, let alone survive long enough to enter a cell where it could be translated to protein. Second, once the RNA had entered the cell, the amount of protein the cells' factories would produce was far too low.

Colloquially, scientists began referring to the molecule by a telling nickname: "messy" RNA. Many of those who persisted with mRNA were condemned to academic obscurity. Flying in the face of consensus, Uğur and Özlem saw extraordinary potential in this ugly duckling.

"It became clear that mRNA had very specific features which we could leverage," says Özlem. Since all an mRNA drug would contain was lines of genetic code, it could be engineered and produced within weeks rather than months. The relative simplicity of the technology made it easier to isolate antigens, or even minuscule components of antigens—known as *epitopes*—and copy their genetic code into a synthetic mRNA template. Once the strand was introduced into a patient's body, their cells would do the rest of the work.

If—and it was a very big if—*if* they could find a way to bring the mRNA to the right immune cells in the human body and keep it stable and active for long enough, the possibilities were *almost* endless. Replacing the set of instructions carried by a strand of mRNA with their own, custom-made commands, would mean that they could just hijack a naturally occurring mechanism and deliver a code that let the patient produce their own drug. They wouldn't need to introduce potentially toxic pharmaceuticals into the human body. The couple aimed to take the code that produced distinctive molecules on cancer cells and simply deliver them to the immune system's army barracks. The body would then use the information to print its own wanted poster for the immune system's sharpshooters.

Uğur and Özlem's passion was not shared by the wider scientific community. It seemed mRNA was destined to spend many years in the scientific desert. The prospect of any respected regulator allowing clinical trials of an mRNA drug to go ahead were slim, especially as most pharmacology experts lacked a detailed understanding of how the molecule went about its business.

While they never gave up on the mRNA technology, Uğur, Özlem, and their academic research team worked on a plethora of immunotherapy approaches, some of which were far more promising, at least in the short term. One of these became the basis for their first business, Ganymed Pharmaceuticals, which focused on developing monoclonal antibodies that can be used to orchestrate a precise attack on cancer cells. The company was extraordinarily successful and ended up being sold for $1.4 billion, in Germany's largest-ever biotech deal.

Yet even those who had invested in Ganymed and saw the couple defy the odds took a dim view of their mRNA ambitions. In 2005, when they mentioned their plan to pursue mRNA therapies to the venture capitalist Matthias Kromayer, the former microbiologist thought the couple had lost the plot. "I was the first to tell Uğur that it was crazy," Kromayer, who had done research into mRNA himself, remembers. "I considered it to be science fiction."

But the doctors and a small group of researchers they had assembled at the Johannes Gutenberg University in Mainz never gave up on mRNA, nor did a handful of other of similarly maligned microbiologists around the world.

By October 2018, when Uğur entered the auditorium of a converted East German cinema in Berlin,[14] the scoffing from the scientific community had subsided. BioNTech, the company he had started with Özlem a decade earlier, had treated more than four hundred cancer patients using mRNA technology, and several clinical trials had been started in Germany, the U.S., UK, and elsewhere. These efforts had come to the attention of Lynda Stuart, an immunologist and director at the Bill & Melinda Gates Foundation. "They were collecting a suite of different approaches, amassing a really interesting tool kit for cancer therapies," she says. Keen to know more, the organization invited Uğur—at the last minute—to deliver a plenary talk at its annual Grand Challenges meeting, an event designed to help solve global health and development problems and attended by dignitaries, including Chancellor Angela Merkel.

Uğur was somewhat surprised to receive the invitation. BioNTech was not in the infectious disease field, he protested, and all he had to present was data showing how the company had used mRNA to prompt a strong immune response to cancer cells. But Stuart's team explained that the foundation often looked at "adjacent" scientific disciplines whose innovations might help fight infectious diseases—especially immuno-oncology, which was beginning to generate a buzz. Gates had recently made an investment in an HIV program that ended up helping cancer. Now, perhaps, cancer could repay the favor and help rid the world of a virus or two. "We were doing a lot of horizon-scanning to see what the trends were, what was changing, who were the cutting-edge people," Stuart says, "and BioNTech clearly surfaced."

Wearing a somber gray suit and open-necked, light-blue shirt, Uğur began his speech at the meeting in Berlin by recalling how much it had pained him, as a physician, to tell cancer patients that their time was almost up. "Why is it that, every year, billions of dollars are invested in cancer research, and yet, for most patients with advanced cancer, cure is the exception, but not the rule?" he asked, while Özlem watched from home on a livestream. After a pregnant pause, he delivered the punch line. "The answer is that cancer drugs do not address the root cause of cancer failure." Every patient, he explained, "has a different cancer . . . composed of billions of diverse cells. The drugs we offer patients today ignore this complexity, ignore the *plasticity* of the disease."

The way to address this, Uğur continued, lay in replacing largely ineffective, off-the-shelf drugs with tailor-made medicines, in which the mutations that are unique to each cancer patient would be targeted. An initial clinical study, pioneering BioNTech's individualized mRNA vaccine in skin cancer patients, had shown promise, he told the conference. Then, at the end of his twelve-minute presentation, Uğur offered a teaser.

Each of the individualized RNA vaccines that his company was making was a race against a patient's rapidly growing tumor. "The vaccines have to be produced in a few weeks," he said in his accented English, and BioNTech had developed the technology to do so. One day, this technique could be "useful for rapidly spreading infectious diseases, so that a vaccine can be delivered in time." mRNA held the key to simpler, safer, and faster drugs that could be deployed against a new virus within days of its discovery.

In the panel discussion that followed, Tedros Adhanom Ghebreyesus, the bespectacled head of the World Health Organization, who would go on to become a prominent figure in the fight against COVID-19, was effusive in his praise for BioNTech's "very encouraging" cancer breakthrough. "I was even saying to Bill [Gates] that this could be the next Nobel Prize," he said.[15] The billionaire responded by hailing another German mRNA company, CureVac, in which his foundation had already invested, as a "huge pioneer." Later that afternoon, however, Uğur found himself in a stuffy hotel room, making his case, face-to-face, with the world's biggest philanthropist.

More than two years later, on that weekend in late January 2020, as he did the math and realized that a new killer virus was rapidly spreading around the world, Uğur's mind kept going back to the discussion he'd had with Gates.

The Microsoft founder—who, rather ironically, loathes PowerPoint presentations in what he calls "learning sessions"—had asked for advance briefing documents, in which Uğur had explained how BioNTech amassed an arsenal of tools, all under one roof, that could be used in combination to stimulate various parts of the immune system and might be useful in the fight against knotty infectious diseases, such as HIV and tuberculosis. Gates had clearly read the files carefully. He pleasantly surprised Uğur, who had ditched his jacket, with a series of quick-fire questions that evinced a deep understanding of the subject matter.

"It was fairly technical; Bill always enjoys the technical," says Stuart, who was in the room. At one point, struggling to explain a cellular principle, Uğur stood up, marched across the room to a flip pad in the corner, and "drew something about 'AND' and 'NOT' gates—a formula from digital logic," Stuart recalls. "It was about how you can target something to a cell using binary coding." The performance appealed to Gates's software expertise. The immune system, he was being taught, could also be hacked—and one of the world's best biohackers was standing right in front of him.

An hour-long discussion about BioNTech's different technologies followed. Gates, who had just lost an old friend to cancer, seemed impressed. Had he known of Uğur's experimental therapies earlier, he said, he would have been in touch. He quizzed Uğur on how BioNTech was able to run clinical trials for cancer drugs, given how small the pool was of people at a particular stage of the disease and in a particular location. But the billionaire's most burning question was whether Uğur's team had given much thought to infectious diseases. Was there potential, he wondered aloud, to develop mRNA-based drugs, in record speed, during a pandemic? Uğur might want to consider preparing a "plug-and-play" solution for that moment, Gates said, as a matter of urgency.

After that pep talk, BioNTech expanded its infectious diseases pipeline, collaborating with Pfizer on a flu vaccine, with the University of Pennsylvania on various pathogens, and with the Gates Foundation on two of the "big three" infectious diseases that ravage the developing world: HIV and tuberculosis (the third being malaria).

But at the time Uğur first pondered the possibility of developing a coronavirus vaccine, in January 2020, those projects had barely started and were far from being ready for clinical trials, let alone regulatory approval or rollout. The mRNA doubters may have toned down their taunting, but the hurdles to getting an entirely new drug class accepted by mainstream medicine remained as high as ever.

Nonetheless, Uğur heard a call to action. For almost thirty years, he, Özlem, and their team had devoted themselves to developing drugs that would tackle cancer, a far deadlier and much more complex menace than this new coronavirus. They had studied the immune responses that evolution had perfected over millions of years to fight pathogens, including viruses. They had engineered mRNA platforms to redirect these responses against tumors. Now, these tools were ready to take on another threat. "In a crisis, unconventional solutions often get more attention from decision-makers," Uğur had told BioNTech chairman Helmut in his discussion on that January weekend. In this emergency, mRNA drugs could come to the rescue. Particularly if, as Uğur was beginning to believe, the coronavirus proved to be a comparatively easy target.

Viruses are spectacularly harmless on their own. They need to enter a cell to reproduce and have developed extraordinary powers of molecular deception to do so quickly, evading the immune system in the process. Traditional vaccines tried to thwart this by introducing a similar or less severe version of the pathogen into the body, which the body recognizes as an invader and will remember to repel when it encounters the real thing—ideally, before the virus has a chance to latch onto unsuspecting cells. But building such products is a delicate and, most importantly, time-consuming process. By contrast, all an mRNA-based vaccine would have to contain was a single strand of genetic code, easily synthesized in a lab with widely available materials, to prompt the body to produce a small part of the virus on its own. The immune system would then deploy its entire arsenal against this foe and, with any luck, be prepared for future skirmishes.

First, though, Uğur was forced to embark on a coronavirus crash course, about which he knew relatively little. The basics were easy enough. Since the 1960s, when human coronaviruses were discovered, seven types have been observed. The first four are seasonal and cause the common cold. The next two, SARS and MERS, caused increasingly severe respiratory diseases and claimed hundreds of lives, before fading from view. The last one was the novel coronavirus, soon to be named SARS-CoV-2.

Learning about the structure of coronaviruses was a harder task. A quick search on academic portals returned several hundred papers on the subject; far too many to be consumed that weekend. The terms used to refer to coronaviruses also varied, making it difficult to get a comprehensive picture of the research to date. Uğur started sifting through dozens of the most relevant studies, his browser cluttered with a dizzying array of tabs. Meanwhile, as Özlem sifted through résumés for potential BioNTech recruits and prepared for her upcoming speech at a university in the Austrian Alps, Uğur happened upon a slew of studies on the first SARS virus, against which several teams had attempted to develop a vaccine. Their efforts hit the buffers once the virus disappeared, pharmaceutical companies lost interest, and funding dried up. But researchers had made one big advance: they had provided a crucial clue that the coronavirus family could be beaten by science. Better yet, they had identified a potential target for vaccine developers.

The clue, it turned out, was in the name. Coronaviruses were so called because of a set of spikes on their surface, which vaguely resemble the prongs on a crown, or *corona,* in Latin. These bulbous proteins, which are roughly twenty nanometers in length[16]—small enough that fifty thousand of them can fit on a pinhead—would soon become a familiar sight, used in virtually all visual representations of SARS-CoV-2. They were what made the virus such a menace—coronavirus spikes could bind to a specific receptor on healthy lung cells and infect them. But they were also the invader's Achilles' heel. In theory, the immune system could be taught to disable or disfigure the molecular protrusion, thus interfering with the docking process and rendering the coronavirus harmless.

To figure out how much this new virus shared with the 2002 SARS virus, Uğur looked up the genetic code for the pathogen, which had been sequenced by a quick-thinking Chinese professor just a couple of weeks earlier and posted online. Never one to trust a single source of information, he cross-referenced the sequence with updated versions that had since been uploaded to public servers. It showed that the Wuhan pathogen was roughly 80 percent similar to the SARS virus, suggesting the spike protein would still be the best target for a vaccine.

Merely identifying a target, however, was not enough. Vaccine development, Uğur knew, hinged on precision. If BioNTech was to design a drug that reproduced the spike protein outside of its natural context, it had to be flawlessly configured, an exact copy. Otherwise, the immune response induced by a jab would fail to recognize the real virus when confronted with an infection in the real world. The vaccine's wanted poster had to perfectly portray the felon—a badly sketched facial composite would not do.

It was by no means a given that an "artificial" spike protein, made in a lab, without the rest of the virus's particles that keep it stable, would share every microscopic dent and divot with the spike as presented on a coronavirus in the wild. Being off by a fraction of a hairbreadth might not only render a vaccine useless but could also even endanger those who received it. Understanding this risk, Uğur pored over the genetic sequence and a digital model of the virus he had quickly generated, looking for precise points in the chain at which he could "splice" the protein, while keeping enough of the surrounding letters—known as *amino acids*—to stabilize it, so that it retained a perfect shape. The precise chemical makeup of the DNA was also important. The sequence, Uğur found, was full of A-U pairings, a constellation that would make it difficult to design a vaccine.

Wherever he looked, Uğur told Özlem when she came back from a run, there were several unknowns.

The couple knew they could not afford to devote their time to another pet project. Uğur's presentation at the J. P. Morgan conference, just days before, had barely mentioned infectious diseases, and BioNTech's shareholders, whose patience had already been tried with twelve loss-making years, were hoping to see several cancer breakthroughs in the coming months. Now, without knowing much about this new virus, a team would have to be assembled that would choose which part of the coronavirus to isolate, what type of material to wrap the mRNA in, decide how large the doses should be, and whether to experiment with a single-shot vaccine or one that was coupled with a booster. If the jab ended up causing illness, allergic reactions, or induced a weak immune response, they would have to walk back every single step and work out what had gone wrong by process of elimination. The risks were enormous.

But Uğur and Özlem also knew the race against the virus was already on and that every week would count. They did not want to be left wondering, "What if . . . ?" On January 24, 2020, there were fewer than a thousand confirmed cases of the new disease internationally. By the twenty-fifth, Uğur and Özlem had privately committed to making a vaccine. By Sunday night, the twenty-sixth, Uğur had designed eight different vaccine candidates and sketched the technical construction plans for them.

The first case of SARS-CoV-2 in Germany would be confirmed the following day, when a thirty-three-year-old worker at a car parts supplier in Bavaria presented with flu-like symptoms at Munich's specialist infectious diseases and tropical medicine institute.[17] By then, BioNTech would have begun a project that would involve deploying hundreds of staff and spending millions of euros to develop a vaccine using an unproven platform against an as-yet unnamed threat.

PROJECT LIGHTSPEED

Radios were important to the Şahins. Every weekday evening, having returned from his tiring shift on the production line of the Ford plant in Cologne, Uğur's father, Ihsan, would fiddle with the antenna on a small wireless, until the hiss and crackle from its tinny speakers gave way to a muffled Turkish folk track. The variety program by Ankara Radio in the early 1970s, along with a beloved record collection, were among the family's precious few connections with a home they had left in search of economic opportunity.

Much to Ihsan's irritation, though, the shortwave signal in West Germany—transmitted from three thousand kilometers away—was not very stable. At a local secondhand shop on his way home from work, from which he had bought the household's gramophone and a sewing machine for Uğur's mother, Ihsan purchased several radios in the hope that they would improve the sound quality of his favorite station.

The beat-up devices were in constant need of repair. "On the weekend, I would watch as my father spread out his tools on the kitchen table," says Uğur, "patiently trying to fix appliances that were generally the worse for wear." It was a torturous process for young Uğur to observe. Like many kids, he fancied himself an engineer and longed to get involved. Uğur vividly remembers excitedly barking instructions at Ihsan, a loving but stern man who believed that children should be seen but not heard. "My father, of course, ignored my instructions and did what he thought was right," says Uğur, recalling the frustration of those childhood hours, "and I only got my chance when he got stuck." Reluctantly, after he had exhausted his own attempts, Ihsan would silently follow Uğur's suggestions. The radios would buzz back to life.

As he cycled to work on the Tuesday morning after he had made the decision to dedicate a significant chunk of his company's resources to building a coronavirus vaccine, the memories of his father and the radios came flooding back to Uğur. "People," he had discovered back then, "have to convince themselves." As a teenager, Uğur's discovery of this precept was reinforced by the critical rationalist philosopher Karl Popper, whose works he stumbled upon during hours spent browsing the neighborhood bookshop while his mother visited nearby department stores. Popper believed that the way one arrives at what can be called "truth" is by submitting bold and imaginative hypotheses to the "tribunal of experience."[1] If a suggestion or an idea survives attempts to refute it, such as Ihsan's attempts to exhaust all other available options with his screwdrivers, one is left with a corroborated fact. "I learned to be patient," says Uğur, whose brain would often be galloping ahead of those he was seeking to persuade, "and be confident that reality would win the day."

On any other week, that principle was a sound one to live by. It had served Uğur well as a physician, a researcher, and a venture-capital-dependent entrepreneur. But pedaling hard on that overcast morning in January (Uğur had given up trying to get a driver's license when he realized how much time car owners wasted sitting in traffic), Uğur knew this was one occasion on which he could not afford to wait for others to come around to his way of thinking. The statistical projections he had toyed with over the weekend were unequivocal. A global pandemic was on its way, and none of the nonclinical methods—be they handwashing, mask-wearing, quarantines, or lockdowns—would be enough to stop it. A vaccine might, but *only* if it arrived in time. Uğur needed his fellow board members—waiting to start their weekly meeting at BioNTech's gleaming headquarters—to share his sense of urgency. *Every single day,* Uğur thought, as his blue-and-silver mountain bike zipped past the famous stained glass Marc Chagall windows of Mainz's gothic Stephanskirche, *really counted.*

That case would be hard to make. During Uğur's fifteen-minute commute, reports were coming in confirming that the number of cases in China had risen by seven hundred in a day, to almost three thousand, and European countries were organizing repatriation flights for their citizens stranded in Wuhan. Germany's blue-chip stock index, the DAX, opened almost 1.5 percent lower, over fears that the virus would hurt companies, like the national carrier Lufthansa, that did a lot of business in China. But only fifty or so cases had been identified in the rest of the world. Health minister Jens Spahn had told the press in Berlin that Germany was "well prepared" to deal with the virus. The head of the Robert Koch Institute, the country's health agency, had sounded similarly sanguine when interviewed on national TV just days earlier. "On balance, we do not expect the virus to spread very much around the world," he had said,[2] when asked what he made of this strange disease. The atmosphere was not one of undue alarm.

Entering his sparsely furnished office at eight o'clock, Uğur saw no signs of panic on the faces of the three executive board members who had gathered around the large white table. Exhausted from the J. P. Morgan conference in San Francisco and the meetings that followed, their minds were already half focused on the upcoming winter break and ski trips in the Alps. The trio had prepared for discussions on the proposed acquisition of Neon Therapeutics, the Boston-based start-up Uğur had visited on his U.S. marathon, and on further fundraising to meet the costs of looming clinical trials for cancer drugs. But instead of sticking to the prepared talking points, Uğur began the meeting with a phrase that the managers in front of him had come to recognize as ominous, "I've been reading . . ."

After Özlem, who had walked to work to rack up Fitbit steps, joined the meeting, Uğur recounted his weekend's research, from stumbling upon the *Lancet* article to mapping Wuhan's transport routes. In the last couple of days, he added, more crucial information had emerged. The coronavirus, it seemed, had a two-week incubation period,[3] making asymptomatic spread even easier. "If someone presents with pneumonia to a European hospital today," he told the room, "no one would consider them to be suffering from a SARS-like disease." Before any doctors realized what they were dealing with, that patient would infect several others. This new pathogen was an invisible enemy at the gates and was probably already in the immediate proximity of the campus on which they were gathered. Uğur let the board in on the macabre projection he had made on Sunday evening—humanity would soon be faced with its first out-of-control pandemic in decades. Then he told them what he had been doing since coming to that conclusion.

Twenty-two hours earlier, the very same room had been a hive of activity. While Özlem was away delivering her guest lecture in Innsbruck, Uğur had summoned leaders from most of BioNTech's departments, as well as the company's few infectious disease experts, to the office he had deliberately placed amid a row of labs, so that he could regularly pop his head around the door and shoot the breeze with BioNTech's technicians. In back-to-back meetings, he briefly repeated his findings and told them of his snap decision to develop a vaccine against the virus that had emerged in China.

The revelation hardly came as a shock. BioNTech staff had become accustomed to receiving an annual "January surprise" from Uğur when they returned after the Christmas break. With more time to think over the holiday period, Uğur would focus exclusively on a narrow topic—often one that had been leading the company to a dead end. In 2018, for example, a melanoma drug had induced a great immune response in human trials. But for some reason, only a fraction of patients' tumors actually shrank. The weapons were being manufactured, but they weren't always firing with sufficient power. In the new year of 2019, having read all the related literature of the last few decades and having discussed findings with Özlem in their weeks off work, Uğur presented a potential solution: a modified molecule that supercharges the sharpshooters of the immune system, to be used in combination with the aforementioned drug. He immediately dedicated a team to the new project, to the mild annoyance of some managers. "Quite often, we would start new projects, and that new project was always the hot project, until it was not," Sebastian Kreiter, one of the most senior scientists at the company, remembers.

This time, Uğur made very clear, was different. His latest project was not about testing a new idea, it was about execution. The company would use *all* available resources to respond to the outbreak of an infectious disease in real time, starting that day. Over the weekend, he told those huddled in his office, he had already made a start. He informed them of the eight possible coronavirus vaccines he had sketched plans for, based on BioNTech's existing mRNA platforms. Each had a different chemical or molecular design and target. But that was just a fraction of the potential combinations. He asked the company's cloning team to cast their eyes over the constructs, and "come up with more suggestions to complement them." Then he asked those responsible for testing a potential vaccine on animals to design and prepare studies, and mRNA experts in charge of manufacturing to get ready to produce more clinical trial material than they had ever produced before. "We *have* to become a vaccine production company," he said. A more detailed plan would come together in the next few days, Uğur added, but for now, each of them was to go back to their departments and get the ball rolling as a matter of priority.

Like Uğur and Özlem, the company's senior managers were hardly expert epidemiologists. But they all knew that previous attempts to take an entirely new vaccine through the drug development process in time to stop a pandemic in its tracks had failed, by wide margins. The sequential steps they would need to take to get BioNTech's first-ever drug to market were almost impossible to accelerate, some protested.

First, they would need to complete an enormous amount of preclinical work, including designing the vaccine and testing it on cells in a lab. That step alone could take several months. If the results were encouraging, they would then embark on studies that would determine if the vaccine worked in mammals and whether it was toxic to rodents. In the unlikely event that rats got severely ill or died, BioNTech would be forced to start from scratch with a new design. There was no way to expedite this step—known as a *toxicology study*—it took half a year to design the experiments, get approval from authorities, compile the necessary paperwork, and monitor the animal subjects up close.

Armed with positive data from such preclinical studies, BioNTech would then be able to apply for authorization to test its candidate on humans in clinical trials. The company would have to run a Phase 1 study involving just a few dozen healthy volunteers, merely to assess the right dose and whether the vaccine caused dangerous side effects. A Phase 2 study would follow, in which a few thousand participants would be assessed. Then a Phase 3 global study would be required, involving tens of thousands of participants from a range of age groups, ethnicities, and geographies, to ascertain the effectiveness of the vaccine. Even for the deadly Ebola virus, where efficiency was built in to the vaccine development process, these clinical stages took almost four years to complete. At any point during this prolonged and expensive procedure, the coronavirus vaccine could fail, either by not producing an immune response or by causing serious side effects. BioNTech would have to go back to the drawing board.

But Uğur had saved his big reveal for the end. To up the chances of producing an effective vaccine in time, he said, BioNTech would completely rewrite the vaccine-maker's playbook. The company could not afford to test a prototype, discard it if it didn't work, and repeat the process over and over again. Instead, it would embrace a strategy that Uğur, frustrated by how long it took to develop cancer medicines, had been mulling over for a while. "We can't put all our eggs in one basket and test just *one* vaccine candidate," he told those crowded into the small room, which was beginning to resemble a bus terminal, "we must build and test *multiple* vaccines in parallel." In normal times, drug development was a bit like walking through a garden labyrinth, until, after reversing out of several dead ends, you emerged into the light again. Faced with a looming pandemic, Uğur said, BioNTech would speed things up. It would send several designs into the labyrinth of preclinical studies and move forward with the first to make its way back out again.

The lineup would be rigorously tested in the lab, on animals, and eventually on humans. At any stage, those contestants that were found not to be safe enough or effective enough would be discarded. At last, a winner would emerge. There would be no time to improve those that disappointed or wait for promising stragglers to catch up. The first out of the labyrinth would become *the* vaccine.

It was to be another six weeks until the World Health Organization declared the coronavirus outbreak a pandemic and four months until Donald Trump's White House launched its Operation Warp Speed vaccine development program. So far, there were no reports of anybody outside China dying of the disease. But by the end of that same Monday, BioNTech had begun working on what would, in the space of eleven months, break every modern record for the production of a medicine. The company, at Uğur's urging, "would go as fast as possible within the laws of physics." With a superhero-movie fan's sense of the dramatic, he had already come up with a name for this historic mission. "We'll call it," he said, standing at the whiteboard and spelling out the words as he spoke, "Project Lightspeed."

Uğur did not need to do much to convince his scientific colleagues in those Monday meetings. But the following day, as he relayed this bold plan to his fellow board members, Uğur sensed he had not yet won over the room. While Özlem, the company's chief medical officer, had taken his prediction seriously, British chief commercial officer Sean Marett, who had been the first outsider to join BioNTech's board in 2012, questioned the wisdom of worrying about a pathogen that was still five thousand miles away. "My response was, 'This is in China; why do you think that's going to be a problem?'" says Sean. "It seemed so distant; it was just a blip on the horizon." Sierk Poetting, BioNTech's tousle-haired chief financial officer, and Ryan Richardson, an American investment banker who had been promoted to chief strategy officer weeks earlier, also had their reservations.

Clearly, Uğur had some persuading to do. He did not *want* to be forced to summon images of bodies piled high to persuade the rest of the board of his argument. But he needed them to understand that such apocalyptic scenes were, at best, just weeks away. If he waited to be vindicated by reality, à la Popper, it would be far too late.

With this in mind, Uğur walked over to a whiteboard and began to sketch a crude version of a graph that would soon become a familiar sight at government briefings the world over, one that showed the number of infections rising exponentially along a sharp curve. "I remember he said, 'This is going to go everywhere,'" recalls Ryan. "He said, 'It is going to be a problem for Europe, for the United States, and for our company,' meaning our employees. I thought: 'Wow, that is very specific.'"

Uğur proceeded to provide a history lesson on the speed and trajectory of pandemics. Even if things didn't look too bad right now, he stressed, they might very soon. In April of 1918, he said, the first wave of the so-called Spanish flu was not much more lethal than the seasonal variety. Although it did spread with alarming rapidity among troops deployed in the First World War, most of those who succumbed to the disease were either elderly, frail, or very young. A far deadlier wave followed between October and December, caused by the treatment of those with severe disease in hospitals, who then infected doctors and fellow patients. An estimated twenty million people died in this three-month period, including a huge number of twenty-five to thirty-five-year-olds.

Mercifully, there was no clear indication as yet that the Wuhan virus was dangerous to healthy youngsters. The vast majority of the few dozen fatalities reported in China were older than sixty-five, and many suffered from preexisting conditions, such as diabetes or hypertension. But just a few days earlier, authorities in the Hubei Province revealed that a thirty-six-year-old man, who was otherwise in fine fettle, had died just two weeks after being admitted to hospital where he had been treated with antivirus medication and antibiotics.[4] This, Uğur warned, might be the canary in the coal mine. In the evolutionary race between viruses and their human hosts, pathogens constantly change their configuration, attempting to sneak past existing antiviral defenses.[5] The coronavirus was not particularly destructive at present, but it could suddenly mutate and turn on the young and fit.

In another horrifying scenario, the virus could become even more efficient and infect more people, much faster. "Everything would be over in just three months," Uğur said, with morgues overflowing and the global population decimated long before a vaccine could be built in the lab, let alone produced or distributed. *Every day mattered.*

If the coronavirus outbreak had happened two years earlier, BioNTech's board would not have entertained the idea of building a vaccine. But thanks to recent improvements to its technology platforms, Uğur was convinced that the company had the tools to respond to a pandemic. Creating mRNA vaccines with its proprietary platforms was now possible, and if delivered in time, its coronavirus shot could come to the rescue long before a traditionally made vaccine. "I think," Uğur said, "we should go all in."

BioNTech, however, was no longer a start-up. After going public in October, it had to consider how such a pivot would look to the outside world. Prioritizing a coronavirus vaccine would undoubtedly delay some of its ongoing cancer programs. "There were some people in the room who were skeptical," says Ryan of Uğur's proposition, "who thought that it would be a distraction." In the eyes of American fund managers, BioNTech was not an infectious diseases business. "We had really good momentum on the share price," says Ryan, who was afraid of spooking shareholders with the announcement of an expensive scheme to tackle a threat that no one else was taking too seriously. "Investors thought we were a pure-play oncology company." BioNTech, which had accumulated more than €400 million of debt in eleven years, needed to raise more money soon. Failing to reach its stated goals would make that all the more difficult.

If the company rushed headlong into a coronavirus vaccine project and didn't succeed, "it could have been the end for BioNTech," fellow board member Sean says. Since the listing on New York's Nasdaq in October, the board was obliged to take minutes of meetings, which could be obtained in the event of a challenge to the company's corporate governance. Under the German legal system, all board members were equally liable for costly missteps.

Then there was the risk of reputational damage. BioNTech had come this far by talking up the potential of its technologies. A coronavirus vaccine program would create a lot of buzz for the mostly unheard-of company, but the odds of it failing or taking too long were far from insignificant. Many of the critical tasks ahead—from running large clinical trials to manufacturing large batches of a pharmaceutical—had never before been attempted by the company, let alone at the speed and scale that would be required to beat a pandemic. If Project Lightspeed turned out to be a damp squib, "it could become a very difficult situation for our company," Özlem acknowledged in that board meeting. "On the other hand," she added, "a full-blown pandemic would anyway be a threat to our people and the company." Why wait for others to guide the world out of this looming crisis if BioNTech had the capability to do so itself? "Shouldn't we," Özlem said, "at least make an effort?"

For a few seconds, the room fell silent. While this decision required a leap of faith, ultimately, the trio to whom Özlem had addressed the question were all there because they trusted her and Uğur's instincts. They had not joined BioNTech to say no to big ideas.

Sean had been working for a small biotech and was on the hunt for commercial partners in 2003 when he met Uğur, who talked him through a suite of technologies he thought could cure cancers. "I just thought this is going to be one of the big ideas of this century—I really thought that," he remembers.

Ryan had been working in health care finance for J. P. Morgan and was on the team that executed the sale of Ganymed, Uğur and Özlem's first business. He got to know the couple, and, when BioNTech began preparing for an IPO, or initial public offering, they asked him to come on board. Ryan had turned down many similar requests from other organizations, but this was "a different category," he says. "It was so ambitious, right from the beginning." He left what was a plum job and hitched his horse to the couple's wagon.

Sierk, a physicist by training, had been working as a management consultant for McKinsey & Company when he was asked to advise the Strüngmanns—the Bavarian billionaires who ended up backing BioNTech—on the sale of their former company. In 2007, Helmut Jeggle, who went on to manage the Strüngmanns' investment vehicle, told Sierk he had "found the Genentech of Europe in Mainz," referring to the wildly successful American biotech that had joined the ranks of Big Pharma. Soon after, Sierk met Uğur at a bar in Munich, and the two spoke for hours. "The way Uğur tells the story of his science, you think: 'Oh, it must work,'" he says. Sierk had always wanted to be an astronaut, to be involved in a moon shot project. This, he felt, was his chance.

Sean, Ryan, and Sierk were won over by Uğur. As long as they could limit the amount spent on the coronavirus program in the next few weeks, during which they would get a clearer picture on how quickly the disease was spreading and how well the vaccine development was progressing, the risks, they felt, were worth taking. "Uğur is normally right," says Sierk, "so we thought: 'Let's support him.'" The board would continue to monitor the situation and could pull back the reins if they felt it necessary. Unanimously, they gave Project Lightspeed the green light.

As everyone sipped their now-lukewarm coffees, the discussion turned to practical matters. Individual roles and responsibilities were clear from the start. Sierk would handle supply chains and production capacities, and manage the war chest. Sean would lead talks with companies whose help BioNTech might need. His merciless negotiating skills would be important in forging any potential collaborations. Ryan would prepare to communicate the entire strategy to the financial markets when the time was right. As well as overseeing the scientific work, Özlem would prepare for clinical trials.

For his part, Uğur was chiefly concerned with "eliminating idle periods." There could be no pause in the Lightspeed teams' early experiments, he said. Shifts would be put in place to ensure round-the-clock work. Then he proposed a four-step approach, to begin immediately. Step one was to prepare for essential preclinical tests—in labs and on rodents. Step two was to get a team in place to design human studies and identify part-ners that could help BioNTech run such trials worldwide. Step three was to expand manufacturing capacity to ensure the company could supply a vaccine to anyone who wanted it. Step four was to prepare for the com-mercialization of the world's first licensed mRNA drug. Uğur had already instructed his staff to start step one the day before, on Monday. "Step two is going to start today, if everyone agrees," he told the board. "Step three will be really, really expensive," he said, "but if we want to make a differ-ence, we have to start it very soon."

Next, Özlem addressed the question of how many of BioNTech's 1,200 employees to devote to the task. "If a full-blown pandemic hits," she argued, "our cancer trials won't be able to continue at full pace, in any case." Freeing up people for a coronavirus vaccine project might make sense. "Having something useful to work on while the world goes into paralysis," she said, "may be a blessing."

No matter how many staff were seconded to the Lightspeed team, there was a limit to how much BioNTech could do in-house. The company had just enough talent and resources to complete the first steps of this am-bitious program. It had experience of carrying out Phase 1 and Phase 2 human trials for cancer drugs and had developed strong relationships with contractors who helped them run such studies. But, while clinical trials involving those with a particular form of late-stage cancer were complex to organize, the number of healthy volunteers involved in tri-als for a preventative vaccine would be orders of magnitude higher than those included in all the studies BioNTech had done to date. Since 2012, it had administered its mRNA drugs to just over four hundred people. The coronavirus shot would need to be tested on *tens of thousands.*

The company would also need to apply for commercial authorization in several countries. This mammoth task would entail preparing supply chains and distribution networks, building a sales force, drawing up lit-erature for patients and health care providers, and much more besides. BioNTech, which, before the coronavirus struck, was still years away from a licensed drug, had the sum total of a single staff member responsible for commercialization. It had no experience at all in sales, marketing, or media relations.

For a moment, the board considered building up such capabilities. After all, the company's long-standing aim was to become a fully integrated bio-pharma business, one that did all the cutting-edge research and also brought its innovations to market. Quickly, "we realized we could not do it alone," says Sean. It would take too long, and speed was paramount. Project Lightspeed would need help from a larger corporation.

Over the years, BioNTech had entered several research and development partnerships, including with European pharma giants Sanofi and Roche. But only one of its well-established tie-ups focused on infectious diseases—the collaboration to develop an mRNA flu jab, which BioNTech had signed with Pfizer in 2018. The U.S. corporation had shown a keen interest in the evolution of the technology and might just be tempted to join forces on a coronavirus project, if only to discover whether this new drug class could be useful in future outbreaks. Pfizer was the obvious first choice.

After instigating Project Lightspeed on Monday, January 27, Uğur quietly approached Holger Kissel, a molecular biologist who had moved into business development at BioNTech after spending much of his career in New York. Holger had been involved in the negotiations that led to the flu partnership with Pfizer and had developed a rapport with the company's management. Would he, Uğur asked, set up a call with Phil Dormitzer, Pfizer's chief scientific officer for viral vaccines and a vice president at the American group, to gauge his interest in a further collaboration?

Soon after, Holger sent an email relaying the request. The subject line read: "Wuhan coronavirus."

At 3:30 p.m. on Tuesday, soon after the board meeting, Uğur jumped on the call Holger had set up with Phil. After exchanging pleasantries, the U.S. executive moved on to the matter at hand. "Guys," Holger remembers Phil saying, "this is not going to work." An industry veteran, Phil had worked for Novartis, where he had led the Swiss group's response to influenza pandemics and had been involved in discussions about whether to create vaccines for the SARS and MERS viruses. Both pathogens had been contained by public health measures before any such projects got off the ground, and Phil believed the same would be true of SARS-CoV-2. "My working assumption was that it would be controlled," he says. Also, experience had taught him that vaccines *always* come too late, even with established technologies. Phil, an RNA expert himself ("That was one of the reasons Pfizer hired me," he says), had been one of the driving forces behind the flu deal with BioNTech and was familiar with its toolbox—and its limitations. The company's mRNA platforms had never been used in clinical trials for infectious diseases, he pointed out, and there was no evidence to suggest it could outpace a pandemic. Uğur recounted the arguments he had presented to others within the company over the previous forty-eight hours. Politely, Phil agreed to think it over. A few hours later, however, he sent an email to say that he had discussed the proposition with other Pfizer colleagues, who agreed that BioNTech's technology was simply not mature enough to take on this challenge.

More than a year later, I asked Uğur how he dealt with this rejection, just hours after the launch of the most important project of his professional life. "*Disappointment* is the wrong word," he says. "Phil's assessment was completely rational, given his experience, and I understood that we couldn't do anything to convince Pfizer at that point." The lessons learned while watching his father, Ihsan, fiddle with radios in the 1970s echoed in his mind. It was only a "matter of time," Uğur thought, before the large pharma company, faced with a global health crisis, would change its assessment. Karl Popper had taught the young Uğur that reality would win the day, eventually. The outbreak in Wuhan, he remained convinced, fulfilled all the criteria for a pandemic.

Undeterred by Pfizer's refusal, Uğur began to focus on the next task on his list: dealing with regulators.

He had managed to mobilize a team to begin work on several constructs at once, accelerating the only part of the vaccine development process that was entirely under BioNTech's control—the preclinical stage. He had tried and, so far, failed to persuade a large corporate partner to help with the final stage, the large-scale clinical testing and licensing of the drug. But that could wait. The more pressing problem was the preparation for the interim stage—administering an entirely unproven vaccine to humans.

If Project Lightspeed was to even get off the starting blocks, the regulators would need to be on board from the get-go. They would have to work with BioNTech to compile a checklist of safety requirements for clinical trials, which the Lightspeed team could tick off before the first needle entered the arm of a healthy volunteer.

The regulation of mRNA drugs had slowly evolved in the decades since Uğur and Özlem had first turned their attention to the molecule. Back in the late 1990s, nucleic acid drugs—those based on DNA or RNA—were still broadly defined as "gene therapies" by the U.S. Food and Drug Administration, or FDA, and by the European Medicines Agency, or EMA. This was a category that became the subject of hysterical commentary by anti-vaccination voices, who sometimes compared emerging therapies to the creation of Frankenstein's fictional monster. Scare stories abounded about genetic engineering leaving a permanent imprint on patients, after observations of DNA-based vaccines had shown that some did end up modifying—albeit harmlessly—the existing genome.

In truth, messenger RNA, which the body degrades within minutes of it fulfilling its function, can do no such damage. The molecule only ends up below the outer perimeter of human cells and is highly unlikely to alter DNA. Regulators, including Germany's Paul Ehrlich Institute, or PEI, were aware of these characteristics. Since 2012, when the BioNTech team dosed their first cancer patient with a first-generation mRNA drug, Uğur and Özlem had spent hundreds of hours presenting to the PEI, and authorities in various countries. Thanks to their close collaborations with these agencies, the company's trials expanded rapidly, with severely ill people receiving BioNTech therapies in studies across Europe, North America, and Australia.

By the time the couple decided to devote their efforts to a coronavirus vaccine in 2020, there was still no internationally harmonized set of requirements for approving mRNA drugs. But in the United States, and particularly in Germany, the groundwork had been laid.

In the late 2000s, Germany's national regulator, the Paul Ehrlich Institute, inadvertently found itself at the heart of an mRNA research cluster. The organization, named after the Nobel Prize–winning immunology and chemotherapy pioneer, had two young companies under its watch. CureVac, founded in 2000 in Tübingen, in southwest Germany, and BioNTech, which came along eight years later in Mainz, were at the forefront of mRNA research worldwide and were eager to test their technologies in humans. Despite having a reputation for being more cautious and conservative than its American counterpart, the PEI had been instrumental in developing a regulatory framework for mRNA vaccines. Over the years, it worked with the start-ups to ensure the molecule was safe to administer to humans. Its staff even coauthored scientific papers[6] with mRNA pioneers, including Uğur and Özlem. The couple attended "research retreats" organized by the regulator—essentially workshops during which the frontiers of medical research were discussed in detail. The innovators and the regulators learned about novel technologies, such as mRNA, together.

Although the bureaucratic obstacles for starting clinical trials on its home turf were higher than in other countries—not least because of strict and decentralized ethics committees—BioNTech continued to run a significant portion of its cancer trials in Germany, in no small part due to the working relationship it had with the PEI. The regulator knew the mRNA scene and could be counted on to take sudden advances in the field seriously. Uğur had developed a collegial relationship with its leader, the biochemist Klaus Cichutek.

On that Tuesday, soon after meeting with BioNTech's board, and before speaking to Pfizer, Uğur picked up the phone and called Klaus directly. He urgently needed to book a scientific advice meeting with the PEI's panel of experts so that, together, they could align on a vaccine development strategy and design a checklist for the Lightspeed team to tick off in the weeks ahead. This would consist of requirements considered essential by PEI for clinical trial authorization, including how lab tests and animal studies had to be run and what quality control measures would need to be in place to ensure manufacturing of the pharmaceutical was up to a consistent standard. In normal times, it would take at least three months to get an appointment to talk through such issues. Uğur needed to get to the front of the queue immediately.

In his conversation with Klaus, Uğur stressed that he was taking the coronavirus outbreak extremely seriously, that BioNTech had initiated a vaccine development program, and that it had pulled staff off other projects. "We want to do this as fast as possible," Uğur remembers saying. "But first, we need feedback."

The regulatory chief, who had worked on DNA and vector vaccines, was not surprised by the request. "It was a natural extension of the work that had been done before," Klaus says of BioNTech's vaccine plans. An early champion of experimental therapies, Klaus promised to do what he could to help and said that he would "look for an available date" for a meeting. "This was not a special service for Uğur," he says. The PEI was already providing emergency advice to other drugmakers and had waived its administrative fees for all coronavirus requests. Uğur did not let on that he would be seeking to move at a much faster pace than even Klaus was imagining. With the "goodwill" of regulators, Uğur had told colleagues, needles filled with an approved, safe drug could be going into arms around the world by the end of the year. This, he warned, would be "pushing the limits of what is possible."

Two days later, on Thursday, Klaus called back. PEI's expert panel might be able to make itself available for a meeting by the end of the following week, he said, so long as BioNTech was able to send a detailed briefing dossier outlining its vaccine plans a couple of days in advance, to give the institute's employees a chance to pore over the details.

Compiling the document Klaus required, the Briefing Book for Scientific Advice, was a complex task at the calmest of times. It involved a comprehensive rundown of every aspect of a potential drug's development, from the underlying technology to the raw materials and active ingredients that would be used, to the precise designs of preclinical safety studies on mice and primates. Normally, this would take between four to six weeks to complete. BioNTech had less than five days and was starting from scratch. It would have to move faster than it had ever done before; indeed, faster than anyone in the industry had ever moved.

There was only one person at the company who could make this happen. Corinna Rosenbaum had joined BioNTech less than two years earlier. She was the lead project manager on its flu vaccine collaboration with Pfizer and had organized the presentation of that case to the PEI in 2019. A specialized research and development coordinator, Corinna would be able to pick the right people to join the team leaders who had already kicked off Project Lightspeed, ensure they were all communicating properly, and keep an eye on the budget. On Thursday, January 30, Uğur sent her an email: "Can you be in my office in ten minutes?" To his surprise, he received no response.

Corinna was at home, enjoying her first day off work, after she had reduced her hours by a fifth to spend more time with her two-year-old son. Busy with mealtime, she was not aware of Uğur's message until she checked her phone a couple of hours later, only to be greeted by a flurry of missed calls and emails marked as important. When she rang back to find out what was going on, she was told that, given her experience pitching a prophylactic, or preventative, vaccine to regulators, Uğur wanted her to lead the company's charge against the novel coronavirus that was racing through China. Corinna had barely heard of the pathogen's existence, bar a few snippets from news reports and the occasional online news story. But the prospect of being at the forefront of a medical breakthrough was too exhilarating to pass up. "It was like a movie situation where the music starts to play," she says. Within minutes, she replied to Uğur's email, saying she was "ready and up for the task" and would be in his office the next morning.

At 9:00 a.m. on Friday, Corinna found herself at the white table in Uğur's office, along with a dozen BioNTech managers. Still in his cycling gear, Uğur delivered his well-rehearsed explanation of how the data predicted a rapid spread of the coronavirus and how, although it seemed strange to suggest this while the general public was untroubled, an enormous death toll was inevitable. The cancer company Corinna had joined was about to be transformed into an infectious diseases juggernaut. The immediate hurdle, however, was the Paul Ehrlich Institute, which was ready to meet on Thursday—six days away. "We need scientific advice in a matter of days," Uğur said, referring to the briefing dossier for the expert panel. "It needs to be a communal effort."

Most people think of regulators as staid organizations that enforce a set of directives and rules with no wiggle room. But behind the faceless façade of these official bodies are hundreds of scientists, whose years on the benches have taught them that scientific advancement does not happen within neatly defined categories. The process of petitioning for clinical trial approval begins, even at the most conservative of agencies, with open dialogue. Just like in a courtroom, experts such as those at the PEI are always free to interpret their "lawbook," so long as they are presented with a convincing argument, supported by scientific data.

Corinna, playing a similar role to an advocate in front of a judge, would have to ensure that BioNTech's best case was put forward. The fifty-page briefing document, finessed by Özlem, would claim that the company had the materials, technology, and expertise to create a safe and successful pharmaceutical. Moreover, the booklet and the discussions that followed would ultimately need to persuade the PEI that the risks of forging ahead with a clinical trial for a group of untested mRNA constructs were outweighed by the benefits of a coronavirus vaccine.

There was one immediate hurdle for Corinna to consider. To ensure that the precious molecular cargo in BioNTech's coronavirus vaccine was delivered to its cellular destination, it would have to be encased in a unique chemical wrapper. But the company had never before used this formulation for injection into a human muscle.

Wrappers had been essential to ensuring mRNA vaccines saw the light of day. In the 1990s, when Uğur and Özlem were experimenting with the technology, its main drawback was the molecule's vulnerability—when outside its natural cellular habitat—to attacks by the body's own enzymes. Strands of mRNA synthesized in a lab could be injected into humans in their "naked" form, but the vast majority of the payload would be instantly degraded, with only a select few survivors making it all the way to the targeted cells. When Sebastian Kreiter had injected mRNA directly into lymph nodes of mice in the early 2000s, almost 99 percent of the molecules were lost. As a result, enormous doses had to be administered to elicit any immune response. In 2012, BioNTech's first trial using naked RNA, in which the molecule was injected directly into lymph nodes, was conducted with doses of up to 1,000 micrograms—more than thirty times the 30 micrograms that would eventually be used in the coronavirus vaccine.

There was no doubt about it—for mRNA drugs to be viable, they needed to be shielded as they traveled through the body to find a cell. Soon, a solution arrived on the scene. Microscopic globules of fat known as *lipid nanoparticles* had been used since the 1990s to insert DNA into cell cultures. They had never been used in humans, but early experiments found that, by using just four simple ingredients, lipids could, if formulated correctly, wrap themselves around mRNA and protect the molecule until it reached cells that function as key communicators in the immune system. Crucially, through careful chemistry, lipids could do all this work without provoking an immune attack against themselves.[7]

Over the years, BioNTech had developed its very own lipid formulations, using generic, unpatented models. The company's team of lipid experts grew by the month. In a major breakthrough, they succeeded in creating particles that were safe and effective for use in intravenous drugs.

Lipids that directly enter the bloodstream are particularly tricky to design. They travel around the body in an instant and can prompt an allergic reaction that leads patients to suffer anaphylactic shock. More importantly, such particles make a beeline for the liver, a dangerous place to prompt an immune response. But by 2014, BioNTech had become the first organization worldwide to use lipid-enveloped mRNA, delivered intravenously, in a clinical trial. The formulation helped the mRNA enter lymphoid tissue, areas of the body where the snipers of the immune system congregate in large numbers, waiting for orders to deploy. Thanks to this advance, a dose of 50 micrograms was sufficient to achieve a robust immune response[8]— twenty times lower than the naked RNA with which the company had experimented two years earlier.

The lipid was useful for cancer treatments in hospitals, where therapies would be administered via a drip, but was less than ideal for a prophylactic coronavirus vaccine intended to be given to billions of healthy people worldwide, in all sorts of makeshift environments. For such a purpose, a jab into the arm was the only workable option. BioNTech had been working on intramuscular lipids, but they had not been a priority and were not yet clinically vetted. The process for producing them, in a clean room, had not been developed and would take too long to put in place. Instead, Uğur and Özlem's team needed a more advanced solution, a plug-and-play lipid that had already passed the muster of regulators, to present to the Paul Ehrlich Institute.

Soon after the nanomedicine world discovered the protective power of lipids in the early 2000s, several companies began to devote themselves to perfecting the chemistry of these unique delivery systems. BioNTech had worked with many of these specialists and tested their formulations one by one. But a tiny Canadian company, with just twenty-five people on staff, had outpaced all its rivals. Acuitas Therapeutics was led by Tom Madden, an English scientist who had worked on lipid formulas in the organic chemistry unit of a firm that suddenly eliminated his position following a takeover. Bruised, Madden took his science elsewhere and, in 2009, founded a start-up in Vancouver—already a hotbed of lipid innovation.

The biotech's formulation was more potent than many others; it was able to deliver mRNA safely and increase the amount of protein—in the coronavirus vaccine's case, this would be the spike protein—created by cellular factories. Most importantly for the regulators, however, Acuitas's lipids were already being used in human trials. The fatty envelopes had caused no harm to patients, nor had they elicited any severe side effects. "It was a remarkable coincidence," says Madden. "We had this really exciting clinical data for a vaccine, at exactly the time that people were becoming aware of the threat from what was to become known as COVID-19."

Although procuring proprietary lipids would come at an enormous cost to BioNTech, pledging to use this familiar design would no doubt ease the minds of PEI's expert panel. If a coronavirus vaccine was to get through clinical studies in less than a year, one thing was certain: Acuitas would need to be on board.

As luck would have it, BioNTech had been in dialogue with the company since 2018, about using its products for a plethora of next-generation, mRNA-encoded antibody drugs called *RiboMABs*. In pursuit of this goal, a team in Mainz had already screened Acuitas's lipids and had all the necessary safety data on hand. Moreover, through these discussions, Uğur and the team knew that Acuitas's lipids were already in the hands of a family-run contract manufacturer in Austria called Polymun, one of the only companies in the world that had developed the niche expertise to combine the precious product with mRNA at a moment's notice. Situated on the shores of the Danube, just outside Vienna, the company was only an eight-hour drive from BioNTech's headquarters. Although the prospect of travel restrictions within the EU seemed ludicrous at the time, Uğur thought it a distinct possibility, within weeks. In such an event, Polymun had the advantage of being close enough for a refrigerated delivery van to shuttle back and forth, if vaccine material was needed urgently for toxicology or efficacy studies.

In the meeting on Friday, Corinna learned that her team would have to convince Acuitas to supply large amounts of its trial-ready lipid formulation, known as ALC-0315, to BioNTech before other manufacturers reserved all the available product. This would not be an easy task, as the company's existing mRNA customers would no doubt fret about intellectual property leaking to BioNTech. Plus, an enormous down payment would probably have to be made to secure stock. But the boss's orders were clear. That same evening, one of the Lightspeed staff emailed Acuitas's Tom Madden, asking to speak to him as a matter of urgency.

Over the weekend, Corinna corralled data from the newly established Lightspeed team for the PEI dossier, including analysis of the mRNA platforms, early details of the potential manufacturing process for clinical trials, and the designs of a toxicology study. Not everyone was up for the task—staff with family commitments or on the verge of burnout politely bowed out—yet the core group had come together within hours. Özlem worked through Sunday night to do her part. The missing piece was still Acuitas, who had not yet consented to the use of their lipids. Then, on the morning of Monday, February 3, Tom Madden offered his help.

By Tuesday evening, a rough version of the briefing dossier was complete. There was no time for cosmetic changes, such as matching font sizes or paragraph alignments; Corinna and a colleague flicked through it to catch serious factual errors. At around 6:00 p.m., just six days after Corinna received the first call from Uğur, they uploaded it to a secure portal on the Paul Ehrlich Institute's website.

On Thursday morning, February 6, a seven-seater cab pulled up outside BioNTech's headquarters to pick up Uğur and Özlem. Inside was Corinna, as well as jet-lagged Acuitas executives Tom Madden and Chris Barbosa, who had flown in from Vancouver for the occasion. The driver, Parviz Zolgharnian, got out to hug Uğur, whom he had ferried around ever since he and Özlem were working at the university hospital in Mainz. Now in his seventies, he was a reassuring presence, one who was there for both the doctors' successes and their failures. Having driven Uğur and Özlem to the PEI's headquarters dozens of times, he knew something important was brewing. He said nothing, but gave them both an encouraging wink.

As they sped along the motorway toward the sleepy town of Langen—just a few miles south of Frankfurt's airport—Uğur pulled out his smartphone and urged his fellow passengers to huddle around the screen. After being reminded by Özlem to wear his seat belt, he played a few seconds of harrowing footage filmed by a Chinese reporter inside a hospital in Wuhan, in which dead bodies wrapped in white cotton sheets were piling up along the corridors. The video provided more evidence for his hypothesis; the coronavirus was far, *far* worse than Chinese officials were letting on.

At 10:00 a.m., the party arrived at the Paul Ehrlich Institute's gray, postmodern headquarters. They were ushered past an enormous bust of the institute's eponymous scientist and into a meeting room, where several other BioNTech team leaders were already seated along one side of an oval oak table, formally dressed. Opposite them were ten of the regulator's most senior decision-makers, each with their own unique field of expertise, including toxicity, pharmacology, and manufacturing. Some of the faces were familiar, having worked closely with Uğur and Özlem on getting other products into the clinic. "We all shook hands," Corinna remembers. "It was one of the last occasions we did that."

First, there was a presentation by Uğur, wearing, unusually, an ironed shirt for the occasion. Pushing a USB stick into the projector, he flicked through slides—in English, for the sake of the Canadian guests—outlining BioNTech's basic strategy for building a coronavirus vaccine, involving three different mRNA platforms and several different dosages. The experts agreed with the concept, but wanted a full set of safety and immunogenicity data to be generated for each vaccine candidate. Next, Andreas Kuhn, a biochemist who had become BioNTech's in-house manufacturing expert, presented the proposed strategy for mRNA production. The PEI experts, who had witnessed the development of the company's plants over the years and had overseen the establishment of quality checks, waved the plans through. After a presentation by Tom Madden, the experts were also satisfied with the lipid formulation from Acuitas. Özlem, who was presenting the plan for clinical studies, hadn't had much time to prepare her part of the presentation. The BioNTech team watched nervously as she took hold of the clicker, but her speech also received a positive reception from the panel. The meeting, despite being prepared in record time, was on track to be a complete success. There was, however, one remaining point of contention—not about the design of clinical trials but the safety precautions with which they would need to comply.

The most time-consuming element in the early stages of vaccine development is a toxicology study, in which a drug would be tested on dozens of mammals—usually mice or rats—to establish if it is harmful. A final report from the study would be needed before any human trials could kick off.

The process usually takes at least five months, and it was this sequence Uğur was desperate to speed up. Days before he sat down to read the *Lancet* article in January, USA's Moderna, the most celebrated mRNA company in the world, announced that it had teamed up with the National Institute of Allergy and Infectious Diseases, an American government agency run by Anthony Fauci, to develop a coronavirus vaccine. Moderna, Uğur had since heard from friends, would not be required by U.S. regulators to run a toxicology study, since it had already tested the same formulation for another vaccine in 2019. The biotech would be able to proceed straight to clinical trials.

BioNTech, conversely, had no such data for the combination of mRNA and lipids it intended to use in a coronavirus vaccine. While the individual components had been tested independently in other trials, they had never been tested as a complete construct. In such a case, regulators would usually require companies to complete a fresh toxicology study with the candidate that was to be injected into humans. But Uğur and Özlem knew that the PEI had significant leeway. If presented with a compelling proposal, it might just err on the side of leniency.

Like all regulators, the PEI had one overriding mission, which had guided its officials through most of the past hundred years, with the exception of a dark period during which the Nazis had attempted to erase the legacy of the institute's Jewish founder. The principle was: "Do no harm."

It hadn't always been this way. After the creation of the first vaccines in the eighteenth century, scientists were free to create and immediately administer experimental treatments with virtually no oversight. Then, after a series of vaccination disasters in the early 1900s, in which shots were accidentally cross-contaminated with other viruses, Western governments began to license and control development and production. Regulations were further strengthened after the infamous "Cutter incident" in 1955, when a batch of polio vaccines ended up giving forty thousand American children the disease. The time it took to get a drug to market slowly increased from months to years.[9]

Germany's lead agency carried the weight of a more harrowing history, commemorated by a memorial outside its entrance. The horror of medical experimentation carried out on prisoners during the Holocaust prompted the establishment of the Nuremberg Code in 1947, which mandated that human trials always be entirely voluntary, be based on safety data accumulated in animal testing, and that the risks to patients should never exceed the potential benefits. These guidelines were built on in subsequent international declarations. They decreed, among other things, that trials be randomized and participants be kept in the dark about whether or not they had received a placebo.

Such conventions underpinned the cautious approach taken by the PEI, the FDA, and others in the late twentieth century and came into sharp focus during the AIDS epidemic of the 1980s and 1990s. The "do no harm" principle, campaigners seeking access to experimental treatments argued, should also apply to the harm caused by blocking access to prospective drugs that could save lives.[10] It was a debate that would resurface a few months into the coronavirus pandemic, when therapies such as dexamethasone, used to treat Donald Trump after he was infected, showed promise in early studies, but were not made immediately available to patients.

Modern regulators, including the Paul Ehrlich Institute, no longer saw their role as simply ensuring that the hazards of drug development were reduced to an absolute minimum. Instead, they would make a series of value judgments, to strike a balance between risk and reward. Some judgments were relatively easy: permanent hair loss, for example, was probably a price worth paying for a successful cancer treatment. But most of the time, these assessments were far more complex. Several attempts had been made to formalize the methodology behind such decisions, but ultimately, it came down to a group of experts in a room, weighing up the options.

The process was not foolproof. In 2006, a cancer treatment was developed by a German company called TeGenero, a spin-off from the

University of Würzburg, just ninety miles east of BioNTech's head-quarters in Mainz. The drug showed no indication of toxicity in ani-mal studies,[11] but caused serious illness within hours of administration to human trial participants and in some cases led to permanent organ failure.[12] Ten years later, a drug designed to treat anxiety and chronic pain, tested in Rennes, France, on behalf of a Portuguese biotech, led to the death of one volunteer and the hospitalization of six others. The product, which worked by breaking down neurotransmitters, had also presented no ill effects in animal tests.[13]

Both of these experimental drugs interfered with biological processes. Vaccines, especially mRNA ones, do not—they work by mimicking natu-ral infection. But what regulators learned from the catastrophes was that toxicology studies did not show the full picture. Soon after, they intro-duced the Minimal Anticipated Biological Effect Level protocol, or MA-BEL. Instead of starting human trials with the highest dose thought to be safe, companies testing a new or risky drug class were mandated to start with the lowest dose proven to prompt a response, based on calculations from in vitro and animal studies. All such trials would start with a single volunteer who would act as a "sentinel" and would be monitored before others could be injected.

The likelihood of a toxicology study for BioNTech's coronavirus vaccine throwing up serious concerns was slim, Uğur and Özlem believed. Most of the individual components—including the lipids—had been well tol-erated by humans in other trials. True, the company's mRNA pharma-ceuticals had never been delivered by injection into a muscle, but they had been administered straight into patients' bloodstreams, a process for which safety standards are far higher.

A cautiously designed Phase 1 trial, Özlem argued to the PEI's panel, could reduce the likelihood of harm being done to human volunteers. "To mitigate any potential risk," she said, the clinical trial would start with a very low dose, on a single subject. The vaccinated individual would be kept overnight to monitor potential side effects. The administration of higher doses, or the inclusion of more volunteers, would have to be cleared by a safety committee that reviewed all the available evidence, at every step of the way. A toxicology study could even be carried out in parallel with the Phase 1 trial, which would be paused at the first sign of irregularities in the animals' behavior.

The Paul Ehrlich Institute's panel listened carefully and took copious notes. "There was a lot of openness to change the sequence of a [toxicology] study," says Isabelle Bekeredjian-Ding, a microbiology specialist at the PEI, who was in the room. But the experts did not agree to allow Uğur and Özlem's teams to abandon the normal procedures for such a study. They wanted more data.

Klaus, who had seen his fair share of viral outbreaks, admits that at the time, the PEI was "still unsure" about whether there would be a pandemic. "At this point, we didn't know if this [outbreak] would be a big thing that would entail all world regions, or would . . . just go away," he says, citing the 2009 swine flu pandemic, which was "gone in no time." It was also unclear how dangerous the coronavirus would be, he says. But none of this played a role in the toxicology study decision, Klaus stresses. "It was clear that we had to insist on critical studies," he says, particularly those that would ascertain whether the mRNA vaccine constructs caused damage to organs.

Uğur and Özlem understood, in principle, the position of the PEI experts. Their concern, though, was that the step would delay the start of clinical trials by months. "We were also fully committed to ensuring safety," says Özlem. "However, given our previous clinical experience with mRNA vaccines, we felt that the toxicology study in animals would not tell us much more than we already knew."

Ultimately, the disagreement the PEI experts had with BioNTech was not on the *risks* of an expedited process but on the *benefits*. The quizzical looks on the faces of many of those who sat opposite the couple showed they believed the virus—which did not appear to be anywhere near as deadly as Ebola—would probably be contained. "We saw the same risk for the individual subject," Uğur says, "but thought it was acceptable in the circumstances, if we ran a cautious Phase 1 trial. Their equation was different. They had not yet seen the pandemic uncontrolled."

The PEI's position, Uğur believed, would change once governments and regulators grasped the true scale of the devastation that would be caused by this novel coronavirus. Yet waiting for them to come around to his way of thinking, with the patience he had learned from watching his father's attempt to fix radios, was fraught with risk.

During the influenza pandemic of 1957, for example, an existing vaccine was tweaked within months of the outbreak, saving millions of lives. A decade later, however, when a new strain of the flu emerged in Hong Kong, science came too late. The 1968 pandemic ended up claiming up to four million lives.

A much more recent outbreak had provided a valuable lesson in the importance of speed. In April 2009, a swine flu vaccine program was set up by the Obama administration. Needles started going into arms six months later, and the vaccine prevented roughly 1.5 million cases, according to estimates from U.S. public health bodies. But a report published years later by the Centers for Disease Control and Prevention contained a damning statistic. Had the vaccine been rolled out just one week earlier, the number of cases prevented, it said, would have been almost 30 percent higher. Two weeks earlier, 60 percent. If the program had been able to start *eight* weeks earlier, it would have prevented millions of further infections.[14]

Uğur was unaware of this report when he deliberated with the PEI panel, but had done enough reading over that weekend in January to understand the underlying concept. In this looming pandemic, he said, "weeks will be decisive." There was a short window in which BioNTech could prepare, before Germany was hit by the coronavirus too. "I fear," he said, "that the risk/benefit assessment will change very quickly."

As he spoke, the first U.S. case of what was still being called 2019-nCoV had been identified in Washington, D.C., in a man who had returned from Wuhan a week earlier. The virus was already everywhere, and a vaccine was the only tool left. Sitting in the PEI's boardroom, Uğur wondered whether the outbreak would prove so deadly that clinical trials would be scrapped altogether and an untested vaccine offered to the public to prevent a substantial section of the global population being wiped out.

He thought it best to keep such suppositions to himself.

The discussion with the PEI panel—never heated, always forensic—went on for two hours. Jugs of coffee and plates of small, individually wrapped cookies were quickly depleted. As the meeting drew to a close, the Paul Ehrlich Institute experts said they would maintain contact with regulators in Europe, the U.S., and Asia and closely monitor the situation. Then they asked when to expect an official application from BioNTech for the commencement of clinical trials. The framing of the question left Uğur and Özlem with a sinking feeling. Would BioNTech, the panel asked, "be submitting by the end of the year?"

It was abundantly clear that the PEI was still expecting to work on a vaccine that would be developed within traditional timelines. The panel did not believe, it seemed to the couple, that BioNTech would be able to accelerate the cloning of constructs and the production of clinical material to the point where regulatory hurdles were the limiting factor. Not wanting to shock the PEI experts, the couple gave each other a knowing look and soft-pedaled their response. Özlem promised to be back in touch when the team had a "better understanding of their schedule." What she did *not* say was that BioNTech would be ready within weeks, rather than months.

Uğur was still unwilling to give up hope on being able to adjust the timing of a toxicology study. Before leaving the PEI boardroom, he told the attendees that BioNTech would follow up with a detailed analysis on the safety of the company's proposed constructs and the danger that a coronavirus pandemic posed.

When Uğur was a kid, it hadn't mattered to him that he was forced to wait until his father figured out the best way to fix a radio. In fact, he says, "the relationship became better" once he realized that letting Ihsan get to the right decision on his own was the only effective tactic. But now, when the stakes were at their highest, that approach had been found wanting. Karl Popper was right: reality—in this case, the reality of the coronavirus crisis—would catch up with everyone, including the PEI panel, eventually. By mid-March, when there would be more than two hundred thousand confirmed cases worldwide, regulators from several countries would waive the requirement for a full-length toxicology study for some vaccine technologies. But by then, with the world in lockdown, precious weeks would have been lost. In the cab on the way home from Langen, Uğur set plan B in motion.

"Corinna," he said, "go book the tox study."

3

THE UNKNOWNS

When Uğur arrived back at BioNTech's custom-built campus in Mainz, his thoughts drifted from the rapid development of a coronavirus vaccine to a more domestic problem. His family was due to travel to the Canary Islands in two weeks' time, for a holiday the couple had promised their teenage daughter in 2019, when preparations for the company's flotation had consumed much of their free time. Convincing her, at the last minute, of the need to stay in a gray, overcast Germany due to the threat posed by some far-off plague would be nigh on impossible.

Leaving the country, however, was not without its complications. Already, some BioNTech staff who would be needed on-site had canceled their own time off. Sebastian Kreiter, one of the most senior scientists at BioNTech and a keen triathlete who competed in three or four events each year, had withdrawn from an upcoming race to focus on shepherding the small Project Lightspeed team, and Uğur had praised his dedication in an early meeting.

But Uğur knew that once the scheme was in full swing, it would likely afford him and Özlem precious few private moments, and this short break would have to sustain them, and their daughter, through the turbulent months ahead. In any case, the three holidays they all took each year were, in essence, not much more than a change of scenery—Uğur and Özlem had always used them to catch up on work and get even fitter, via a strict exercise regime, making use of the hotel's running track and pools, with occasional trips to the beach to break up the days. "The truth is, we make a veritable boot camp out of it," says Özlem, and the couple expected to do the same this time, in Spain. The tasks on their to-do lists largely consisted of reading and reviewing scientific papers, making phone calls, and responding to emails, all of which, Uğur reasoned, could be done while catching the last of the winter sun. He would, as usual, insist on paying extra to check in an additional suitcase bursting with electronics, including a laptop and two large monitors, without which he found it impossible to map his thoughts. The family would also bring their own coffee machine and grinder along, ensuring the fuel that the doctors needed for their early-morning work was of a consistent quality. Based on their previous experiences of being contacted by Uğur and Özlem while the pair were ostensibly on holiday, BioNTech employees knew business would continue more or less as usual, regardless of their leaders' physical location.

As for the dangers involved, Uğur argued that until lockdowns were inevitably introduced, there was a higher chance of catching this wretched disease in a local shopping mall than on a beach in Lanzarote. So, after a prolonged discussion with Özlem, the duo decided to head south, regardless. But before they left with their oversize baggage, there was the small matter of BioNTech's biannual agenda-setting meeting, which required their attention.

On February 13, almost all the company's 1,300 staff gathered in the Altes Postlager, an old postal depot near Mainz's railway station normally used for gigs and street food, for a town hall gathering. Once a light lunch was served, chief financial officer Sierk Poetting took to the stage. Against a backdrop decorated with graffiti art, he began to run through a slide deck outlining the former start-up's ambitious goals for 2020, including opening its U.S. headquarters and launching a further nine clinical trials, adding to the eleven already underway.

Thanks to those targets, BioNTech's €300 million budget for the year was being stretched to the breaking point. In fact, due to an increase in spending, and the hiring of roughly two hundred new staff in 2020, the company's finances would soon be back to where they had started prior to going public in New York. If no more money was raised, Sierk said, the coffers would be empty by the middle of 2021. He did not mention Project Lightspeed, which was destined to put further strain on the purse strings. To avoid the team being distracted by a flurry of inquiries, the board had decided to keep the coronavirus scheme secret, even within BioNTech. The company's strategy had always been not to reveal too much during the early stages of a project, and Uğur and Özlem's preference was to do the same when it came to the coronavirus program. The firm's fledgling external communications department consisted of thirty-one-year-old Jasmina Alatovic, plus one new recruit, and the couple wanted to wait until viable vaccine prototypes had been developed before answering questions from reporters, analysts, and investors.

Sierk concluded his presentation, to polite applause, and Uğur walked up to the dais. As the entry music died down, he reviewed BioNTech's many existing programs, from mRNA and antibody therapies to products exploiting the power of T-cells and cytokines. But as was often the case, his slides had not been prepared sufficiently in advance for many others to see them. Over the next few minutes, as employees nibbled on their refreshments, Uğur spilled the beans. He knew that lockdowns were looming and that this might be the last opportunity to gin up excitement among the workforce in person. First, he ran through the science, including a diagram of the four structural elements—the spike, envelope, membrane, and nucleocapsid proteins—that make up the novel coronavirus. Then he summarized the literature on the nature of the disease it caused, which was now being referred to as COVID-19. Two days earlier, the World Health Organization had announced the new moniker in an attempt to replace SARS-CoV-2 in the popular lexicon, a term the agency worried would have "unintended consequences in terms of creating unnecessary fear for some populations" with bitter memories of the first SARS[1] outbreak.

Such tiptoeing was nowhere to be found in Uğur's presentation, which included a stark assessment of global transport routes and the available transmission data for the virus. This pathogen could kill up to 0.3, and possibly up to 3, people in every 100 infected, he told the crowd. The peak of its spread across the globe might not be reached until June. In the absence of effective treatments or vaccines, a pandemic that could cost up to three million lives was around the corner. Given the potential of its technology, the company believed it had a duty, he added, to attempt to tackle the emerging threat.

As I write this in the summer of 2021, with the death toll well over four million, such pronouncements seem eerily prophetic to the point of incredulity. At the time of Uğur's prediction, there were just forty-seven thousand confirmed cases in the entire world, and the disease had not spread beyond the twenty-five countries in which it had so far been detected.[2] The key cause of Uğur's alarm—the discovery that the virus was spread by those who appeared healthy—was still not recognized as a major risk, with the WHO stating that "transmission from asymptomatic cases is likely not a major driver of transmission."[3] Neither Mainz, nor Germany as a whole, felt like places under immediate threat. Angela Merkel's government had recently told the public that their risk of infection remained "very low,"[4] while health minister Jens Spahn dismissed calls for temperature checks[5] on arrivals at airports. But Uğur's warning is there, in black and white, buried midway through an eighty-eight-page presentation, with a small CONFIDENTIAL watermark in the bottom-left corner and the date of the event on the opposite side. It is stated so matter-of-factly that, a few slides later, the deck seamlessly moves on to morale-boosting pictures of staff wearing green company-branded socks with sandals, under the slogan: *BioNTech—as unique as our employees!*

Before those snaps were projected onto a wall in the cavernous hall on that February afternoon, Uğur explained his plan for how the company could marshal its resources to fight COVID-19. He flicked through diagrams of what he believed were BioNTech's most promising mRNA platforms, on which series of vaccine candidates could be constructed. The company had also resolved, he said, to explore if it could use coronavirus-specific antibodies to treat those already infected with the disease. Uğur then introduced those who had already started work on these tasks and asked them to come forward. "At some point," he said, his voice echoing off the exposed brick, "almost everyone in the company may be working on this project." The room began to buzz.

Had Uğur and Özlem been forced to face the public—rather than their own staff—at such an early stage, their responses might not have inspired much confidence. It was increasingly clear to the couple that unless the virus spread so quickly that two-thirds of the world's population were infected within months, a prophylactic was the only permanent solution to the looming global crisis. But they were kept awake at night by a nagging question: What if the virus could not be stopped by a vaccine at all?

There was plenty of cause for concern. Recent medical history provided a catalog of failures, the largest of which were the botched attempts to tackle another deadly virus: HIV. In the decades since it emerged in the 1980s, groundbreaking therapies had managed to significantly reduce the pathogen's lethality, but no vaccine had provided sufficient protection. As its full name suggests, human immunodeficiency virus has the power to suppress the body's immune system, its army of specialized defense units, leaving it vulnerable to AIDS and cancers, among other threats. Frustratingly for scientists, it also mutates at an alarming rate, making it very difficult to identify an antigen, or target, to place on the so-called wanted poster for the immune forces to recognize. There are often more strains of HIV within a single patient's body than the number of flu variants around the globe.[6] Another virus, hepatitis C, which can cause severe liver damage, similarly had thwarted all vaccine efforts to date, even though an effective shot against its "cousin," hepatitis B, had been available for several years. So quickly did the virus evolve that even patients who had recovered from an initial hep C infection were susceptible to a second attack.[7] In addition, vaccines against an array of infections that target the gut, cause acute diarrhea and dysentery, and kill hundreds of thousands of children in low-income countries had also proved to be only partially effective.[8] In short, there were no general rules that could predict whether a particular, newly emerging virus would be amenable to successful vaccine development.

When it came to coronaviruses, the record was not much more impressive. As anyone who has come down with the sniffles in September can attest, scientists have failed to build a vaccine against the common cold, which is caused by dozens of different rhinovirus and coronavirus strains, too varied to be tackled by a catchall drug (although given the mildness of its symptoms, they have not tried too hard). Research had shown that antibodies *could* neutralize the far more dangerous SARS and MERS coronaviruses, but there was no concrete clinical evidence that vaccines worked against them in humans.

Ominous reports were also beginning to trickle out of China and Japan, suggesting that recovered COVID-19 patients who had been discharged from hospitals were presenting weeks later with recurring symptoms. Due to a lack of accurate diagnostics, these rumors were unreliable,[9] and it was impossible to ascertain whether the individuals were merely experiencing a relapse from the same bout of illness. But such dark tales hinted at the *possibility* of reinfection, which, if true, would be a body blow to coronavirus vaccine developers. If convalescent patients developed little or no immunity against the disease, the chances of artificially inducing a durable immune response with a vaccine were considerably lower. Plus, the early data pointed to stark differences in the severity of the disease—some, mostly younger people, developed no symptoms, while others developed fatal pneumonia. Would a vaccine that worked for the first group also protect those that needed it most?

Uğur and Özlem knew that even for pathogens against which an immune response could be artificially provoked, there was a wide range in how effective a vaccine would be. The influenza virus was a familiar enemy, and the mechanisms of flu vaccines had been diligently studied for decades. Despite these efforts, the annual flu jab sometimes offered protection to just over 40 percent of those who received it—nowhere near high enough to stop a pandemic in its tracks. Would a vaccine against the novel coronavirus, whose modus operandi remained a mystery to scientists, be any better?

For now, the Lightspeed team had no answers. In effect, BioNTech would be flying blind for months. It would take until June before they were sure that in most instances the body remembered and repelled SARS-

CoV-2. By the time the first confirmed case of reinfection emerged in August 2020,[10] when a thirty-three-year-old man in Hong Kong was reported to have contracted COVID-19 some 142 days after he first tested positive, it would finally be clear that such incidents were not frequent enough to cause concern. A few weeks after that, Uğur and Özlem would be able to tell the world that a vaccine could prevent severe disease in the vast majority of those who took it. For the time being, Özlem says, the couple "were living with the unknowns."

Yet the question of *whether* a vaccine would work was almost a secondary one. BioNTech, virtually unknown beyond the niche world of biotechnology, was staking its steadily built reputation on a product which could, if not built correctly, do much more harm than good. Once again, there were plenty of precedents for such a worst-case scenario.

In the late 1960s, children in Washington, D.C., received a new vaccine in a landmark clinical trial for the respiratory syncytial virus, or RSV. For most adults, the symptoms of this pervasive virus are relatively mild and similar to those caused by the common cold. But infants infected with RSV—which, like SARS-CoV-2, consists of a single strand of RNA—often develop severe pneumonia and may even die. With millions of babies being hospitalized each year due to the virus, the RSV vaccine was poised to be a significant medical breakthrough. What followed, however, was one of the worst clinical disasters in the pharmaceutical industry's history. Roughly 80 percent of those treated ended up with severe respiratory disease once exposed to RSV,[11] while two children died soon after. Instead of neutralizing the virus, the vaccine appeared to be enhancing its effects. These tragic results perplexed scientists, as the shot contained only an inactivated copy of RSV, which was incapable of reproducing. Some thought that liquid formaldehyde, the substance used to disarm the synthetic virus, was causing the adverse reactions, but the chemical had been used in several other vaccines for years, with no discernible safety issues. For decades, researchers toiled to understand what went wrong, examining tissue from the lungs of the study's participants[12] and comparing the effects of the vaccine on humans to those in mice.[13]

The problem, they eventually discovered in 2009, was that the antibodies produced by the children's immune response to the vaccine failed to properly recognize the RSV. They were clinging on to the perilous particles, but instead of neutralizing the virus, they facilitated its entry into healthy cells.

On that fateful Saturday in January when Uğur sifted through hundreds of coronavirus studies, he learned—to his horror—of similar pitfalls in attempts to tackle the original SARS[14] virus. In 2005, he read, Canadian researchers had built a vaccine using a modified pox virus that expressed the spike protein, that knobby substance on the coronavirus that gives the pathogen its crown-like look and attaches to receptors on lung cells. Then they tested it on ferrets and found that not only did it fail to protect against disease but the animals that contracted the virus after being immunized actually fared *worse* than those in the control group.[15] The same effect ("severe acute lung injury") was confirmed by a team of researchers from Hong Kong who tested a vaccine on Chinese rhesus macaques.[16] Trials on mice and rabbits with a vaccine for the SARS virus's successor, which induced MERS,[17] were also catastrophic.

While scientists couldn't be *sure* about what had gone wrong, they had a strong hypothesis, one that lit up like a large neon warning sign in Uğur's head. When working properly, antibodies were the most potent weapon that vaccines for infectious diseases could coax the immune system into deploying. The minuscule Y-shaped structures would end up binding to the invader—in the case of coronaviruses, to the spike protein—and block it from fulfilling its primary function: attaching to specific receptors on healthy cells and, like a key in a lock, invading and infecting them. But if a horde of these specialized attackers failed to clasp to their target in the correct fashion, their sharp stems ended up helping the virus, by providing an entirely new mechanism for it to break through a cell's membrane. Far from having to rely on binding to a specific receptor, the virus could now attack cells with abandon, using the antibodies' protrusions as an alternative entry route. In other words, if the spears hurled at the assailant were slightly off target, they were picked up and turned back on the body itself.

This phenomenon, known as *antibody-dependent enhancement,* or

ADE, was not new. It had first been reported in the 1960s[18] and was one of regulators' primary concerns when assessing a new vaccine. The smallest of inaccuracies in the design of a new prophylactic could prove fatal. Researchers had spent years trying to sidestep this obstacle, through trial and error. But BioNTech did not have that kind of time. It had one chance to engineer an emergency vaccine before the virus was too widespread to stop.

In discussions with two of his closest consiglieres, Sebastian Kreiter and Mustafa Diken, Uğur had laid out three possibilities. The first, and most optimistic, was that the company would get lucky—its vaccine design, however crude, would not lead to ADE or other adverse effects. The second, and most pessimistic, was that regardless of how hard anyone worked to build a SARS-CoV-2 vaccine, it would end up causing ADE. The third, and most thrilling for the scientific soul, was that a carefully constructed vaccine would eliminate the risk. "We will design different candidates," Uğur said, "perform the experiments, and wait to see what the data tells us."

There was little doubt among the leaders of BioNTech's team about the best way to build a coronavirus vaccine that was both effective and safe—namely, to engineer an authentic copy of the spike protein. A 2009 study had found that the small bulges studded on the surfaces of coronaviruses were chiefly responsible for enabling the pathogens to infect humans. The paper also revealed that the body's *own* immune responses to the SARS coronavirus mainly targeted these proteins, recognizing them as the most efficient way of stopping the threat dead. "We were lucky," Özlem says. Unlike many other viruses, which unfold like a Swiss Army knife, and have a plethora of different-shaped tools for infiltrating healthy cells, "this virus was pretty unidimensional; it had a clear molecule with which it enters lung cells." The Lightspeed team simply had to ensure its vaccines replicated that molecule—in the form of a wanted poster—for the immune system's troops to scrutinize and learn to attack.

To reduce the chances of an ADE disaster, however, the body's forces would have to strike with pinpoint accuracy. The engineered spike—the configuration the vaccine would use to train the troops—would have to match a *particular* shape of the spike as it appears in the natural world.

This was far from a straightforward task. Just before it latches onto lung cells, the spike transforms itself from a thistlelike form into a configuration that resembles a tall goblet.[19] Once attached to the cell, the protein continues to remold itself into a sharp switchblade, with which it pierces through the membrane, fusing the virus and the healthy cell together and allowing the genome to enter and replicate. For a vaccine to work properly, it would ideally be designed to reproduce the goblet-like shape of the spike protein. The immune system's forces would then be briefed to attack the virus before it transformed into the switchblade-like structure it uses to penetrate cells. With any luck, its potent docking mechanism would be disrupted.

For those vaccine companies dependent on deactivating a live version of SARS-CoV-2 in a lab, there was a chance that the methods used to strip the pathogen of its powers, such as applying formaldehyde or extreme heat, could prevent them from perfectly replicating the goblet-like form of the spike. For BioNTech, and those who were hoping to get the body *itself* to reproduce the spike, by providing the genetic instructions to do so, the difficulty was that the protein structure was inherently unstable. There was every chance that when the sequence for the spike—the blueprint for its manufacture—was delivered by mRNA, the human body would end up producing a *slightly modified* structure, rather than the exact one necessary.

If the body's pathogen-fighting forces were not able to recognize the coronavirus properly, a vaccine could prove ineffective. But it could also be dangerous. It was such a scenario that had probably led to the RSV calamity in the 1960s and explained the mishaps with MERS and SARS vaccine prototypes.

Luckily, as Uğur discovered during his weekend research, one man, located four thousand miles away from Mainz, had dedicated his career to stabilizing viral antigens, in the hope that researchers would finally be able to develop effective drugs against RSV, HIV, and others. His name was Barney Graham.

Now a veteran immunologist and virologist at the U.S. National Institutes of Health (NIH), Graham had been raised on a hog farm in Kansas before studying math and eventually turning his attention to biology. After witnessing the devastation wrought by the AIDS pandemic in the 1980s, he developed an obsession with understanding HIV, as well as other troubling viruses such as RSV. Once he became aware of the shape-shifting proteins that were hampering vaccine efforts by making it hard to isolate a target for the immune system's sharpshooters, he set about trying to preserve their form. In 2012, making use of modern bioengineering techniques, he designed an antigen that kept its "pre-fusion" shape, finally raising hopes that a safe RSV shot could be developed.[20]

Soon after, Graham attempted to do the same for the MERS virus, using a sample from a Ph.D. student with flu-like symptoms[21] who had recently returned from the hajj in Mecca, Saudi Arabia—the country in which the pathogen was first discovered. By strategically substituting just two of the amino acids in the protrusion's genetic sequence, he was able to stabilize the spike protein *and* elicit a much stronger antibody response. It was this breakthrough[22] that Uğur read about on that weekend in January and immediately identified as being of potential importance to a successful SARS-CoV-2 vaccine.

It was unclear to Uğur whether Graham had started investigating COVID-19, but the genetic code of the novel coronavirus sequenced in Shanghai had shown that it was about 54 percent identical to the MERS virus; similar enough to make some educated guesses. By further examining the genomes of the two viruses, Uğur realized that Graham's method would probably be able to stabilize the protein in the Wuhan version too. Using this design, the BioNTech vaccines would not only have a much better chance of working well but also of avoiding the dreaded ADE.

Being primarily a tumor immunologist, Uğur had never encountered Graham, whose specialism was infectious diseases. As he investigated, he discovered that Graham was already collaborating with mRNA company Moderna, which had announced, to great fanfare, that it was working on a coronavirus vaccine. But Uğur says that didn't bother him. "I trusted that I could count on a fellow scientist's sense of responsibility," he says. Without hesitation, he sent an email introducing himself to Graham and appealing to the academic's goodwill.

Happily, Graham quickly replied, and friendly exchanges via phone and email followed, in which he and Uğur discussed the available evidence for the configuration of the spike protein in SARS-CoV-2. As it happened, the NIH scientist had indeed been poring over the novel coronavirus's genetic sequence ever since it had been uploaded on January 11. (In fact, he had been one of the prominent researchers pushing for its publication.) In their conversations, Graham freely gave Uğur the information he would need: the molecular equivalent of codes to a locked safe. "I could tell Uğur was a great scientist," says the gray-goateed Graham, whose office is decorated with 3D models of viral proteins. "I just told him what I would do if I was making a vaccine, and that positions 986 and 987 should stabilize the spike."

Graham also waved away questions of a patent conflict with Moderna. "I am a public servant," says the veteran researcher, who has since retired. "The whole reason for doing that is to make things go faster, go better." His collaboration with the U.S. biotech was more conceptual anyway, he says, and there had been discussions at the NIH with the head of its infectious disease agency, Anthony Fauci, about sharing the U.S. government agency's expertise openly if it could aid global efforts to beat the novel coronavirus. "It felt like a crisis, and we had made a decision internally that we would not worry too much about IP or confidentiality," Graham remembers. An exchange between BioNTech's business development team and the NIH followed, and a collaboration was agreed.

The spike protein sleuthing, however, was a long way from being over. As he investigated further, Uğur discovered a rift among researchers.

While many advocated replicating the *entire* spike protein in a vaccine, some believed a better result could be achieved by reproducing just a *fraction* of it, known as the *receptor-binding domain,* or *RBD.* The RBD is the very tip of the spike, the bit that enables it to fulfill its function of clasping onto specific receptors on lung cells. Building a vaccine that only reproduced the RBD would, in theory, make things much easier for many developers. All they needed to do was re-create a *fragment* of the assailant's face on the vaccine's wanted poster, rather than working on a perfect likeness of the *full* spike. Not only would the vaccine be simpler, with less genetic "junk," RBD advocates argued—it would contain just around 200 amino acids, or protein building blocks, out of 1,200 in the full spike— but given the smaller target, the risk of ADE would be significantly lowered. The rest of the spike protein would be untouched by the antibody response, minimizing the chances of errant Y-shaped prongs aiding and abetting the virus. Additionally, the more concentrated the response, the more chance there was that antibodies would neutralize all of the twenty-five to forty individual spike proteins on each invading particle.[23] Aiming at the RBD would prevent the immune system's troops from being distracted by less important parts of the virus and would compel them to focus on what mattered most—blunting the tip of the weapon with which the assailant forces its way into healthy cells.

Among the RBD backers were some scientific heavyweights, notably George Fu Gao, the head of the Chinese Center for Disease Control and Prevention—an Oxford- and Harvard-educated immunologist. Gao and Graham were old friends and had been discussing their varied approaches for weeks. While the American believed his design—using a stabilized full spike—was still the better one, he had gently tried to convince Uğur to build an RBD-focused vaccine instead. "I was trying to help out George Gao," he says. Moderna was going with the full spike, and he reasoned it would be good for the world if someone else tried the alternative option, just in case it proved superior. Little did he know that BioNTech would be covering all the bases itself.

Uğur was drawn to Graham's argument. The receptor-binding domain, he knew, was a "hot spot for mutations," and if, as is normal, variants of the virus began to emerge, it was likely that a vaccine targeting the full spike would remain more effective, for longer. In the world of science, however, hunches are not enough. While both RBD designs and those expressing the full spike had been studied in preclinical tests for the SARS and MERS viruses, they had never been directly compared or benchmarked. There was plenty of convincing literature supporting either side of the debate, but in the matter of Graham versus Gao, there was only one way to pick a winner. The Project Lightspeed team would explore both methods and follow the evidence, in the style of Uğur's beloved empiricist, Karl Popper.

Given the time pressures, such a move was almost foolhardy. Most other COVID-19 vaccine developers had already picked a lane: as well as Moderna, Oxford University had chosen to build its candidate with the full spike, as had Russian and Chinese scientists. But Uğur and Özlem believed that with this virus, weighing up the different antigens, or vaccine targets, could be the difference between success and failure.

Respiratory diseases, they knew, are devilishly difficult to combat. The only opportunity for the immune system's army to ambush airborne particles is during their *millimeters-long* journey from landing on the lining of cells in the nose, mouth, or lungs, to infiltrating them. If a person encounters a high load of the coronavirus, and antibodies are not fast enough, the pathogen pierces through the lining and proliferates within cells, creating tens of thousands—or even millions—of copies. Early publications indicated that the SARS CoV-2 spike protein bound to its receptor with alarming speed and strength, like Velcro, making it even harder for antibodies to neutralize the virus in time. It was *crucial* for vaccine-induced forces to intercept the assailant before it breached barriers.

To address this challenge, the vaccine had to be designed to elicit a particularly strong antibody response. Özlem and Uğur projected that it would probably take two vaccine injections to protect most people from the disease. But the drug needed to do more than just elicit antibodies. To fight back against this coronavirus and avoid repeat infections, the COVID-19 vaccine's antigen—coding for the receptor-binding domain or the full spike—would need to call on *all* the immune system's strengths.

The sharpshooters the body deploys against specific viruses largely fall into two categories. The first line of defense, known as *humoral immunity,* consists of antibodies that attack foreign objects roaming around in our bloodstreams before they have a chance to hitch onto cells. The second wave, *cellular immunity,* deals with those that have slipped through the net. This specialist force, made up of so-called T-cells, attacks and destroys cells that have *already* succumbed to infection.

For some of the most pervasive pathogens, these SWAT teams are surplus to requirements. Rabies, for example, can be defeated by antibodies alone.[24] But to effectively combat the likes of tuberculosis, HIV, and malaria, which can enter and infect cells before antibodies get the chance to neutralize the virus, T-cells are vital. Early studies of recovered SARS patients had shown that these forces had come into play, suggesting that the full immunological arsenal was needed to defeat this new virus too.

The BioNTech team had perfected the induction of such responses when developing cancer therapies, for which T-cells are even more important. They had worked tirelessly on triggering the deployment of two types of T-cells, each with their own powers. CD4 T-cells, also known as *helper cells,* act as early initiators and orchestrators of the immune response. They help other immune cells stay active and have long-term memories, enabling them to recognize a pathogen months, or even years, after being first confronted with the threat. CD8 T-cells, also called *cytotoxic T-cells* (CTLs), have the amazing ability to detect infected cells even when the virus is hidden behind the cell's outer lining. CTLs recognize small fragments presented on infected cells, an ability that gives patrolling CD8 troops the equivalent of x-ray vision, helping them find and kill the enemy, even when camouflaged.

In reviewing the available literature on coronaviruses in January, Uğur had found a study published fifteen years earlier, which demonstrated that CD8 T-cells rendered the SARS virus less lethal. Given that coronavirus's similarity to SARS-CoV-2, the evidence in this paper suggested that a powerful T-cell response would be pivotal when it came to preventing deaths from the novel coronavirus too.

However, bringing too many T-cells to the party was also fraught with danger. Just as antibodies could cause ADE, there was the possibility that these forces would trigger a cytokine storm, in which the immune system goes into overdrive[25] and provokes disease. When deployed accurately, T-cells are lifesavers, but if they arrive at the battlefield a fraction too late, once a virus is already in organs, attacking the "enemy" could cause collateral damage and destroy healthy tissue. In some cases, such a re-action could be fatal. These petrifying prospects "drove me crazy," says Uğur, who compares developing a successful vaccine to briefing a Special Forces unit. If the troops are well trained, they can storm besieged build-ings while keeping civilian casualties to a minimum. However, if they are misdirected or are deployed once the enemy is deeply entrenched, the entire town they are tasked with defending could be destroyed in the cross fire.

The successful recruitment and training of these forces would depend heavily on the choice of antigen, as well as the engineering and delivery of the vaccine's mRNA. With that in mind, the couple spent days draw-ing connections between what they knew of the way the different units in the immune system's army behaved and the available information about SARS viruses. This kind of detective work was deeply embedded in Uğur's and Özlem's DNA. In the heavily politicized world of medical research, where academics are protective of their pet theories, and often bear life-long grudges against those who disparage them, the couple had remained rigidly agnostic, swayed by solid data alone. Here too they would evalu-ate several vaccines, variably using Barney Graham's stabilized spike pro-tein and George Gao's receptor-binding domain antigens. But with each new construct, Project Lightspeed became more complex, and BioNTech needed to hurry.

Uğur had already asked twenty of the company's most senior staff to come up with a plan for the fastest possible development of multiple vac-cines, in preparation for testing them on humans. Unlike in his early meetings with employees in January, there was now more evidence of the emerging threat. The *Diamond Princess* cruise ship had been quarantined off the shores of Japan, with hundreds of those on board testing positive for SARS-CoV-2, providing more proof of the virus's swift spread. Masks were selling out in German pharmacies.[26]

Yet Uğur sensed that many BioNTech experts were still wary of his urgency, and his fears were realized mere days before the couple were due to head off on their long-planned holiday. Uğur had scheduled a team meeting to discuss timelines, but hours before it was due to start, a text message from one of the company's managers popped up on-screen. "Just to give you a heads-up," it read, "they are saying it's impossible to start clinical trials before September."

That afternoon, when Uğur entered his office—jammed with two dozen people—the tension could be cut with a knife. Nervously, the assembled department heads explained that it would be months before they would be ready to start a Phase 1 study. One by one, they went through the steps required to prepare several coronavirus vaccines for administration to humans, including gathering more data on the proposed mRNA platforms, comparing the individual candidates, running a monthslong toxicology study, and producing enough vaccine for the volunteers.

"I hear you, but we have to accelerate," Uğur pleaded with the room. Gently, he insisted on being told *why* each part of the process could not be speeded up. "If you can explain to me that this is not doable by the laws of physics, I will accept that," he said, to the mild annoyance of the senior scientists present, who resented their tried-and-tested workflows being questioned. "He would say, 'But this is how I did it as a Ph.D. student,'" says Stephanie Hein, who would be in charge of cloning the genetic sequences for the vaccine antigens using bacteria, "and we would say, we still need to wait for the *E. coli* to grow!"

In response, Uğur suggested a quicker alternative, which only took a few hours. But once again, his key message was that for there to be any chance of a vaccine beating this virus, the Lightspeed team *had* to complete tasks in parallel. The project's mantra would be "first the fastest, later the best," he said—BioNTech would not be waiting for the perfect construct. All the company needed to do was to ascertain which antigen and which mRNA platform worked best and get the winning vaccine out there. "Once we are in the position to help to contain the emergency situation with a vaccine that protects people and is safe, we can, if needs be, work on an even better second-generation one," he told the room. The priority was to solve the unknowns—whether a vaccine would *work* and whether it would *harm*.

As the discussion continued, it became obvious that answering those questions, via a vastly hastened process, was technically feasible, even if few of those in attendance believed it was possible in the real world. To develop as much vaccine material as possible in-house, to be tested in the lab and on animals, facilities that were normally used for small batches of cancer drugs would be staffed around the clock, Uğur said, although he acknowledged it would be tough to get all external suppliers working at the same speed. His objective for the commencement of clinical research, however, was clear: "We need to start in April."

With these instructions in place, Uğur, Özlem, and their teenage daughter headed off to Lanzarote, computer monitors and coffee machine in tow, making a conscious effort to avoid large crowds. Once they had arrived at their sun-soaked destination, news of the first deaths on the *Diamond Princess* cruise ship began to trickle through, slowly ratcheting up their unease.

As they had expected, however, the doctors' days were consumed by Project Lightspeed, with short, scheduled breaks for running, swimming, gym workouts, or high-intensity training. As well as guiding the teams back in Mainz through the vaccine design process, a proposed partnership with Chinese pharmaceutical giant Fosun that was suddenly gaining pace required the couple's full attention. The conglomerate, which ran two hospitals in Wuhan, had witnessed the outbreak of the coronavirus firsthand and made contact with BioNTech's chief strategy officer, Ryan Richardson, soon after the board meeting in January at which Uğur unveiled his plan to take on this new pathogen. The representative's inquiry had been straightforward: "Are you working on a coronavirus vaccine, and if so, can we speak to you about it?"

Little did Fosun know that they were pushing at an open door. BioNTech's board was already concerned about whether clinical trials—which, to provide useful results, need to take place in an area where some participants are likely to get infected—could be carried out where the virus was most prevalent. "We thought: 'Well, we're going to have to have a partner in China,'" says Ryan, who immediately informed Uğur of the approach. Then, on January 29, Uğur spoke to Fosun's Aimin Hui, a Boston-based executive at the publicly listed company and a fellow oncologist. He found Aimin to be extremely well informed about BioNTech's capabilities, including the results of its clinical trials for cancer drugs. "I noted that they had some advantages over the other leading mRNA companies," says Aimin. "Most importantly to me, they had a diversified platform . . . which would increase chances of a vaccine's success." There was also a sense of urgency in Aimin's voice. His wife had almost been stranded in China a few weeks earlier, due to the outbreak, and told him of the havoc that was being unleashed back home. Unlike many of the decision-makers Uğur was talking to in Europe, Aimin needed no convincing of the threat the world faced.

There were some exploratory talks with other Chinese groups, says Ryan, who had spent a lot of time in Asia trying to make inroads on the continent for BioNTech, but the interest from Fosun "came from the very top." So, just two weeks after the first call with Aimin, Uğur made a quick trip to Boston to meet the executive in person. Their encounter was only supposed to last for a couple of hours, while the two had a light dinner, but "in the end, we talked for close to three hours," says Aimin, "and forgot to eat." The pair sketched the outlines of a plan for clinical trials in China—the epicenter of what was still, increasingly bizarrely, classified as a mere epidemic—on the back of several table napkins. Days later, a confidential agreement was signed between the two companies, enabling an initial exchange of data. While Uğur and Özlem were in the Canary Islands, a more comprehensive research and development plan was drawn up, and an approach was made by Fosun to China's regulatory agency, the CDE.

At 5:00 a.m. on Saturday, February 22, the tired couple found themselves in front of the monitors Uğur had set up in the kitchenette of their hotel suite for a video call with the CDE, in which they were to present Project Lightspeed. With the help of a team formed by Aimin, the doctors had rehearsed their presentation hours earlier, while their daughter read books by the pool. The briefing documents that BioNTech filed to Germany's Paul Ehrlich Institute had been adapted and updated in Mainz, translated by the Fosun team overnight, and sent to the Chinese regulator.

Now, staring out of their screens were a dozen CDE members, in a huge conference room in Beijing, waiting to hear more. The sight with which Uğur and Özlem were confronted was an unfamiliar one to European eyes. The experts were socially distanced, and all were wearing masks. There was no complacency, the doctors realized, among those who had witnessed the devastating effects of the virus firsthand.

On the call with the CDE, Uğur, wearing a business shirt over his beach shorts, explained the company's suite of RNA technologies, pausing every couple of minutes to allow an interpreter to repeat his comments. Andreas Kuhn, in Germany, talked the experts through the manufacturing process. When it came to her turn, Özlem, who was presenting the company's clinical trial strategy, was nervous. "I couldn't read my own slides, as they were all in Chinese characters," she says, "except for an occasional 'BioNTech' thrown in." But a flurry of follow-up questions, translated into English, indicated that she and the rest of the speakers had been well understood. The meeting was supposed to go on for two hours, but "lasted over four," says Aimin, with the Lightspeed team promising to follow up with a list of clarifications.

The very next day, it became increasingly clear that the apocalyptic scenes playing out in China were about to become a familiar sight in Europe. After a third confirmed fatality, Italian authorities had implemented draconian measures to control an outbreak in the north of the country, closing schools and supermarkets and calling off football matches.[27] Then, as Uğur and Özlem sat in their Spanish apartment, ominous reports came in from neighboring Tenerife.[28] One thousand guests and workers at a hotel on the island were forced into quarantine, after an Italian doctor and his wife tested positive for the coronavirus. Concerned by the prospect of health care systems collapsing and infected people being forced to stay at home, putting their families at risk, Uğur began shopping for emergency supplies. "My dad impulsively bought a bunch of stuff on Amazon," the couple's teenage daughter remembers, ordering gloves and full-body hazmat suits in adult and child sizes to be delivered to Mainz.

The family's anxiety was ratcheted up even further when unusually strong Saharan winds hit the Canary Islands, causing one of the worst sandstorms in decades and forcing all airports to close. The trio were due to return home in just a couple of days, but all they could see out of their windows was an orange haze. To their great relief, the weather soon improved, and the holidaymakers' flight back to Germany went ahead as scheduled. Upon their return home, they headed to a local supermarket to stock up on groceries. As they approached the cash register, Uğur and Özlem's daughter made them pause for a selfie to take note of a new fashion accessory. All three were wearing masks.

THE mRNA BIOHACKERS

Sierk Poetting was skiing in the Austrian Alps when the call came. A regional train traveling through southwest Germany, a mildly panicked voice said, had been halted by a convoy of police cars and ambulances outside a small medieval town.[1] Paramedics wearing full-body hazmat suits had proceeded to board the central carriage and emerged propping up a man who looked a little unwell. Hours earlier, according to news agency reports being read out over the phone by a member of BioNTech's HR department, the passenger had flown in from Italy, where he had passed through Milan. On his rail journey from Frankfurt Airport, while trundling along the banks of the Nahe River, he developed flu-like symptoms and, fearing the worst, called a newly established coronavirus hotline. Emergency services were deployed to the scene, where they took down the details of those on board, in case they needed to trace a confirmed infection.

The incident was hardly cause for alarm. It made the local TV bulletins in the state of Rhineland-Palatinate, but did not get much coverage elsewhere. The date was February 26, and although rising rapidly, just four hundred cases had been reported in Italy. The odds of the man on the train having contracted COVID-19 were still extremely low. But the site of the incident, which most Germans would struggle to locate on a map, made the hairs on the back of Sierk's sunburned neck stand up. Idar-Oberstein, hitherto most famous as the birthplace of actor Bruce Willis, was home to BioNTech's largest manufacturing hub, where material for its cancer trials was produced. Already, the team there were exploring whether existing facilities could be adapted to create early batches of a coronavirus vaccine. The epidemic was getting much too close for comfort.

"Okay, that's it now," said Sierk, ending the call. Realizing his holiday was probably over, he removed his goggles and snow gloves and tapped out a short email on his smartphone to members of a crisis task force he had set up soon after the BioNTech board first discussed the novel coronavirus in January. "Let's convene," he wrote, "as soon as possible."

Although nominally in charge of the coffers as the company's chief financial officer, Sierk was also responsible for staffing. Thus far, the health measures he had introduced at BioNTech were confined to a video on the company's intranet (called the *InteRNA,* geddit?), demonstrating hand-washing techniques to the tune of "Happy Birthday," and antibacterial gel placed in corridors. Just a day before hearing the news of the interrupted train journey, the jovial executive had also suggested testing videoconferencing software, much to the bafflement of some middle managers. BioNTech was in the process of finalizing the purchase of Neon Therapeutics, a small cancer medicine company in Boston, and Sierk was convinced that travel between the two countries would soon be impossible. "But," he recalls, "I thought I had a few days."

After discussing the Idar-Oberstein news with the task force, he was ready to go a step further. Trade fairs and sporting events were being canceled across Europe and supermarket shelves emptied of pasta and toilet paper. If one passenger on a local train was all it took to unleash havoc, Sierk thought, a single member of BioNTech's mobile and international workforce carrying the disease could force the company to shut up shop for weeks. While his wife and four boys carried on down the slopes, he began to draft strict guidelines. Anyone returning from a coronavirus hot spot, or living with someone who had recently traveled to such a location, would be banished from the company premises for two weeks.

Uğur and Özlem were firmly in favor of the new rules. They were already concerned that while the Project Lightspeed team were working around the clock to build a COVID-19 vaccine, several other employees had unknowingly attended a potential super-spreader event: the annual Mainz carnival.

The festival, which the couple would flee the city to avoid, was so popular that it was broadcast nationally. Pictures of enormous floats, often featuring ribald caricatures of politicians, would make the front pages, as would images of hundreds of thousands of revelers parading through the streets. It was a fixture few locals wanted to miss. "I went there in my costume—really, it was just like every year," says François Perrineau, who manages the labs at BioNTech. "It was extremely crowded." After the event, François came down with what he thought was "a cold." To this day, he does not know how close he came to being "Patient Zero" in a company-wide outbreak.

On a personal level, Uğur's paranoia had not waned either. Soon after the family returned from the Canary Islands at the end of February, the couple's daughter was reading at home when her mother called. "Sweetie, I am so sorry to hear you are sick," Özlem, who was with Uğur, said loudly and deliberately, to the astonishment of the perfectly healthy teenager. Quickly, she cottoned on that her parents were at an event that had turned out to be more crowded than expected, and Uğur was desperately searching for an exit strategy. "Don't worry," Özlem continued theatrically, "we're coming home to take care of you." A short while later, Uğur burst through the front door and made a beeline for the bathroom, where he lathered soap on his hands and face.

On her morning run, Özlem had taken to listening to a new podcast, featuring a virologist from Berlin's Charité hospital, Christian Drosten, who would soon rise to national prominence. The first episode dropped on the very day that the train passing through Idar-Oberstein was stopped. At the time, Germany had recorded just a few dozen cases and was still sending protective gear and disinfectant to China.[2] Drosten, who was involved in the discovery of the first SARS virus and worked on MERS, was relaxed about people traveling to and from Italy.[3] But he emphasized that with no widespread testing for COVID-19, the true number of those infected was impossible to assess and likely much greater than the official figures suggested. He was clear about one thing: "We do have a pandemic."[4]

As she switched from the podcast to a mix of '80s pop hits that never failed to get her legs moving, Özlem considered Drosten's pronouncement.

When it came to tackling this virus, BioNTech was several yards behind the starting line. Traditional vaccine-makers relying on slower, cumbersome methods had several key advantages. Their platforms had been tried and tested, and hundreds of millions of people had been safely inoculated with drugs based upon them. Existing, fully staffed manufacturing facilities were standing by, ready to produce billions of doses. By contrast, no mRNA pharmaceutical had ever been approved for public use.

Unlike fellow mRNA company Moderna, BioNTech also had no clinical data for the specific combination of their mRNA platforms and the particular lipid wrapper they would use to inject them into muscles. In laboratory experiments, the complex mechanisms that underpinned their innovations had proven to be sound. But it was impossible to predict how they would work in humans and against a pathogen that was largely unstudied. In so many ways, the company was the least likely candidate to create a marketable coronavirus vaccine.

Yet BioNTech, Özlem knew, had a unique advantage. Decades of research had led her and Uğur's teams to a point where the building of an effective vaccine was possible in a matter of weeks. Against the blackest of skies, the stars had aligned. The coronavirus appeared to be a beatable opponent: its spike proteins were clearly defined and not too difficult to disarm. The timing was also fortuitous: in the last couple of years, the company had finally filled their immunological toolbox with mRNA platforms that could give the modest molecule superpowers. It had obtained an assortment of special fatty acid formulations that would protect the fragile mRNA long enough for it to sneak into human cells. Had the novel coronavirus jumped from animals to humans just a short time earlier, none of these technologies would have been ready to be used in a clinical trial. Now, during the worst public health crisis in more than a century, they happened to be in an ideal formation to bring about a medical breakthrough.

To understand the mountain that BioNTech had already climbed and the tools that would help the Lightspeed team reach new heights in 2020, one needs to go back to 1796, when Edward Jenner first inoculated his gardener's son with cowpox, paving the way for modern vaccination.

The method the Englishman used has, in principle, remained more or less unchanged for centuries. Jenner, having noticed that milkmaids exposed to the cowpox virus were rarely stricken by the similar but deadlier smallpox, deliberately exposed the boy to a live version of the former, to protect against the latter. This jolted the child's immune system into action. Crucially, when his body's defenses encountered the enemy in a more dangerous form—smallpox—they would remember the threat and respond in greater force. The concept behind this, while profound in its impact, is technically simple. If the immune system is an army camp, the vaccine is a sentry who bursts through its gates hauling a captured combatant, commanding the idle troops to eliminate this foe, and anyone bearing a resemblance to him, *at all costs*.

Of course, Jenner and his contemporaries did not have a clue about the molecular mechanics behind this procedure. The fields of virology and immunology were yet to be created, and no one would visually examine a virus until the invention of the electron microscope in the 1930s.[5] But the basic technique remains at the heart of most vaccines administered today, even though they contain weakened or fully deactivated copies of a virus or bacteria, rather than live versions. It has helped the world rid itself of smallpox, which killed more than three hundred million people in the twentieth century alone,[6] and has almost eliminated polio and measles.

Traditional inoculations, however, always had their drawbacks. In Jenner's day, the only way of passing cowpox from person to person was by harvesting the infected pus of those afflicted and administering it to others. While effective, this gruesome "arm-to-arm" technique, often involving orphans, sometimes helped spread other diseases, such as syphilis. Later, doctors began to use pus from the skin of animals instead, which, while more practical, did not do much to reduce the risks.

Today, vaccines carry a version of a virus that can be presented to the immune system's foot soldiers in a much safer manner. But to vaccinate a sizable portion of a population, millions of copies of the targeted virus, or one very similar to it, must be made; a delicate and lengthy process during which contamination is a constant threat.[7] In some cases, this is done in petri dishes or flasks, which are then placed in incubators that create the perfect growing environment for the virus, maintaining a constant temperature of 37 degrees Celsius and a precise level of humidity. Mostly, however, the vaccines we have come to rely on to rid ourselves of persistent pathogens are not grown using cell cultures in a lab. Instead, they depend on chicken eggs.

Take the flu vaccine. Every year, technicians at large pharmaceutical companies receive a set of vials from the World Health Organization, containing samples of what the agency believes will be the most dominant strands of seasonal influenza in the coming winter. To create enough material for millions of vaccines, the manufacturer needs to replicate these viruses millions of times over, which is where the eggs come in. A virus is injected into each fertilized yolk, where it reproduces, before being purified by scientists and inactivated, often using extreme heat or disinfectant. The painstaking process is not always successful. Viruses can mutate while growing in eggs, and if they do, they won't perfectly match the flu strains in circulation, limiting the number of vaccine doses.

Aside from being prone to error, the chicken-and-egg system has another obvious limitation, which preoccupied U.S. president Gerald Ford in 1976, when he summoned his cabinet to respond to a swine flu outbreak. His key concern was that the country would not have enough hen eggs to develop sufficient vaccine. The then secretary of agriculture is said to have assured his commander in chief that "the roosters of America are ready to do their duty," but the U.S. has since kept millions of eggs on hand at undisclosed locations, in preparation for a sudden surge in demand during a pandemic.[8] So too have several other developed countries.

This has not helped to speed up flu vaccine production by much. In 2009, when the Obama administration was attempting to tackle a new swine flu strain, it could only move as fast as the reproductive system of poultry. "Even if you yell at them, they don't grow faster," Thomas Frieden, the then director of the Centers for Disease Control and Prevention, told reporters,[9] referring to the rows of eggs. The U.S. had spent billions of dollars on developing alternative vaccine platforms, but none had yet proven robust enough. While physicists at NASA were testing a new telescope that mapped the entire sky every three hours and provided unprecedented insight into dark matter, when it came to pandemics on earth, "the tools that we have available are not as modern as we would like or as rapid," Frieden admitted. It took approximately six months[10] for swine flu vaccines to hit pharmacy shelves, missing the second peak of the disease.

The production of vaccines using the method above has become cheaper in recent decades, and the process refined for maximum efficiency. Some researchers have also adopted an altered technique, creating recombinant protein subunit vaccines, which do not require eggs. Instead of reproducing a whole virus, a fragment of the pathogen, cultivated in huge steel bioreactors, can be introduced to the body's immune troops. But not all fragments are suitable for this approach (which was taken by Novavax and Sanofi, among others, for COVID-19 vaccines), and it often takes months to work out which proteins might be replicable in a vaccine.

Scientists have increasingly concentrated on more promising technologies. After James Watson and Francis Crick discovered DNA's complex molecular structure—the ladderlike double helix that is reproduced in every schoolchild's science textbook—in the early 1950s, the excitement around the molecule helped open a new frontier for vaccines. Instead of introducing a live or lab-grown virus into the body, genetic material could, in theory, turn our cells into factories and direct them to create the protein on their own. The sentry who storms into the army briefing room would no longer need to drag along a handcuffed assailant. He could carry a set of instructions, in the form of DNA, for cells to produce millions of lifelike replicas of the invader—the wanted posters of our earlier analogy. These would then be used as target practice, to train the troops.

Vaccines using DNA, however, largely flopped, and the hype around them initially led only to the development of a few vaccines for animals. Various alternative techniques have been explored, such as the delivering of genetic instructions by wrapping them into a well-known virus, stripped of its ability to do harm, and limited in its ability to replicate. These Trojan horses, so-called viral vectors, were first used in groundbreaking Ebola vaccines and would be utilized by the Oxford/AstraZeneca and Johnson

& Johnson teams, as well as Russia's Sputnik and China's CanSino, to create COVID-19 vaccines in 2020, with varied levels of success.

By the time Uğur and Özlem turned their attention to the coronavirus, however, they were in possession of what they believed to be a far more elegant, versatile, and effective solution, one that promised to finally move science on from Jenner's backyard experiment. It was the result of decades of dedication to incremental advances, with a singular aim: improving outcomes for cancer patients.

The couple's interest in immunology was not originally connected to infectious diseases. As young doctors in the 1990s, they believed that a proper understanding of the immune system might enable them to deploy its sophisticated forces against the cancerous tumors killing their patients.

They were by no means the only ones to come up with this idea. An entire field of *immunotherapy* had emerged, and many devoted researchers were trying (and mostly failing) to achieve the same aim. But as Uğur and Özlem began working together during their early courtship, an immunological revolution was taking place, which would revive the promise of such treatments. The mind-boggling ways in which the immune system organized itself were being revealed in great detail, step by fascinating step. Breakthroughs were being made at breakneck speed. Consequently, nearly two hundred years after Jenner, scientists were starting to understand *how* vaccines worked.

The immune system, it was becoming clear, had, over millions of years, developed specialized weapons, in the form of molecules, and trained specialist troops, in the form of cells, to protect and defend humans against pathogens. During this period, these forces had encountered viruses that employed all sorts of tricks to escape their grasp, but the body had eventually found ways to overcome the wily invaders nonetheless. The emerging understanding of these tactics was opening up a world of possibilities. There was a fully stocked arsenal and a well-trained military *right there* within patients' bodies, Uğur and Özlem realized, which could be repurposed and redirected against cancer cells.

The immune system ignores cancer, which grows within healthy bodies, because it does not recognize it as a danger. Since one cannot predict how tumors will look before they emerge, it is impossible to stop them from growing in the first place by replicating their likeness on a wanted poster in a preventative vaccine. Instead, the holy grail for the couple, and a small community of tumor immunologists around the world, was to harness the powers of the immune system to develop cancer *therapies* that trained the body to recognize existing cancers as a threat and deploy forces to attack and shrink them. These drugs would seek to exploit the same mechanisms as vaccines (and in scientific circles, they *are* referred to as cancer vaccines), but to do so, Uğur and Özlem needed to decipher the complex language of the immune system.

For almost a century, scientists had made occasional breakthroughs that enhanced our understanding of the immune system. They learned, for example, that there were two defense forces within the body. The first, called *innate immunity,* consists of multipurpose regiments stationed everywhere from our skin to our mucus to our organs, who fight all foreign substances they encounter. To continue our military metaphor, these are your standard infantry troops, the germ killers that quickly rally at the site of a fresh cut, for example, and destroy bacteria. The second, known as *adaptive immunity,* contains the sophisticated sharp-shooters we've encountered, the ones that vaccine-makers hope to train to target a particular threat with pinpoint accuracy, such as antibodies and T-cells. It had long been clear that the two forces did not operate in silos. Just as in the regular army, the sharpshooters worked alongside the infantry and coordinated their attacks.[11] But only while Uğur and Özlem were cutting their teeth as physicians in Homburg were researchers finally working out—in a series of quick-fire discoveries—*how* these units communicated.

One of the keys to this newfound understanding was a curious octopus-like structure, first detected in the 1970s by Canadian immunologist Ralph Steinman. In his lab on Manhattan's Upper East Side, Steinman looked through a specialized microscope and identified "dendritic cells," so named because of their many treelike branches. His discovery, which was to win him the Nobel Prize in 2011,[12] was the missing link in scientists' conception of the immune system. Over the next few decades, it became clear that DCs, as they are called in the trade, carry out an array of functions. As "sentinels," they sit in skin and tissues and patrol the body for foreign invaders such as bacteria and viruses. Once they capture an intruder in their tentacles, they transport it to areas of the body in which specialized sharpshooters like T-cells sit polishing their weapons, waiting for a call-up, while B-cells, which make antibodies, stand ready for combat. They are the bridge between the standard infantry of the innate immune system and the sophisticated units of the adaptive immune system.

In the couple's imagination, dendritic cells are the high-ranking generals in the immune army who collect and process information from the environment and from other cells, and use that intelligence to direct troops to strategic outposts. With great fascination, Uğur and Özlem, who had started to study dendritic cells themselves, listened to talks at DC conferences (including ones delivered by Steinman himself) and followed the research of their fellow scientists on the pivotal roles these DCs play in the human body's immune responses.

Armed with a fresh and continuously deepening understanding of how the immune system communicates, cancer immunologists initiated numerous clinical trials. They enrolled patients who had exhausted all standard treatment options and delivered wanted posters depicting newly identified and unique tumor features to the volunteers' bodies, using peptides, proteins, and viral vectors. Academic papers were published showing that some of these methods had indeed triggered T-cell responses in study participants, motivating the couple to continue their research.

But Uğur and Özlem knew that the euphoria surrounding these early results was premature. What many researchers were failing to understand was the intractable nature of their opponent. In contrast to pathogens, cancers are the enemy within. They emerge out of healthy cells and by the time a drug is administered have spread throughout the body, making it hard for the sharpshooters of the immune system to distinguish friend from foe.

The sheer size of the enemy's ranks is also forbidding. Even a small tumor, say with a diameter of one centimeter, consists of up to 1 billion cancer cells. One that has grown to five centimeters already has 125 billion cells, all of which are dividing uncontrollably and growing in number, every single day. Prompting T-cells to join the fight was not enough. "We calculated that the immune responses generated with the cancer vaccine technologies available at that time were too low by a factor of one hundred to one thousand," recalls Uğur. "The immune system's troops were either not mobilized at all by these cancer vaccines or had no chance against the overwhelmingly superior cancer cells, which outnumbered them."

Enormous T-cell armies, the doctors understood, would need to be deployed to successfully engage in cell-versus-cell combat with such a powerful adversary. "We knew that we needed another kind of vaccine," Uğur says. "It had to be much stronger, much more potent, if we were to be successful with this idea."

There was yet another reason to cast about for a better technology. As Uğur and Özlem's research progressed, it was becoming apparent to academics around the world that every patient's cancer was different—too different to treat with a catchall drug. The tumor immunology research community, initially excited about the prospects of cancer vaccines, had to accept the reality that fighting tumors in this way was not as easy as they had hoped. Out of disappointment, an increasing number of scientists turned to other topics, but in their lab in Saarland, Uğur and Özlem dug deeper. "If every cancer is different," they mused, "why don't we develop a vaccine technology that can be tailored to each individual patient's tumor?"

To do this, the couple needed to achieve two things. "One was to find a versatile way of communicating with the immune troops, to inform them about the precise molecular properties of the enemy," says Uğur. "The other was to sound the alarm, underlining that this is information that must be acted upon as a high priority." In practical terms, they needed a way to deliver a message directly to the DCs—the generals—and to inform them in detail about the characteristics of the approaching enemy so that they deployed the immune system's troops in large numbers.

One of Uğur and Özlem's first ports of call was DNA.

Unlike the vaccines that had come before, direct vaccination with DNA meant that proteins—parts used as wanted posters—no longer needed to be produced in cell cultures or in eggs and introduced into the body. Instead, this technology would allow the doctors to deliver nothing more than genetic information—a set of *instructions* to make proteins. If taken seriously by dendritic cells, the instructions could lead the body to create its own wanted posters in the form of proteins that could be used as target practice by the T-cells, which were particularly important when it came to fighting cancer. Uğur and Özlem tested DNA vaccines on mice and were excited by some good early results. But when they tried to repeat the experiment with human dendritic cells, the couple were disappointed.

Because DNA is the so-called hard copy of genetic information, it is normally found deep inside the cell's nucleus, or central core. While rodent cells divide, allowing strands of foreign DNA to enter the gap caused by the split, human cells are not quite as hospitable. The uptake of DNA strands by human dendritic cells, it turned out, was uneven, and inadequate.

The pair soon spotted a work-around. It was based on the central dogma of molecular biology, first dictated by Francis Crick: *DNA makes RNA, and RNA makes protein*. In other words, DNA, which contains a hard copy of genetic information, passes its protein-making instructions to RNA, which takes them to cellular production lines. Synthetic RNA was easy to produce and, as far as the doctors knew, safe. Instead of introducing DNA into a patient, which would then make RNA, which would then command cellular factories to build a protein, or a wanted poster, they could simply cut out the middleman and send RNA on its own.

Even better: messenger RNA, the form of RNA that transports *the actual* instructions from DNA to the cell's production lines, has one simple task, and it does most of its work in the cytoplasm, a large area in the cell where the hard work of protein production takes place, just below the outer membrane, or soft shell. Delivering mRNA to this part of the cell, Uğur and Özlem theorized, would be a whole lot easier than getting foreign DNA *all the way inside* the inhospitable nucleus.

Experiments with mRNA had started twenty years earlier, in the 1970s,[13] primarily as a fact-finding mission for scientists who wanted to get a clearer understanding of how cellular machinery functioned. By 1990, American gene therapy pioneer Jon Wolff[14] discovered that mRNA injected into the muscles of mice was taken up and the proteins for which it encoded were produced. This, he claimed, could provide an "alternative approach to vaccine development,"[15] and soon after, French researchers near Lyon got positive results from a similar experiment.[16] But this disparate group of mRNA enthusiasts were not even on the fringes of the medical science mainstream, and Uğur says that "even within the small community, we were largely ignoring each other." For their findings to have been dismissed, they would have had to be taken seriously. Instead, they were almost completely ignored, and many moved on to other disciplines. mRNA was not even *considered* a viable vaccine class by seasoned immunologists. And with good reason.

For all its drawbacks, DNA can be kept on a shelf for weeks and is fairly robust. Technicians have to wear sterile masks, gloves, and lab coats when working with the molecule, but such basic precautions are normally enough. That is why DNA can easily be recovered by detectives at a crime scene without too much fuss. mRNA, while chemically stable and able to withstand high temperatures, is instantly destroyed by enzymes called *RNAses* that are everywhere: in human hair, breath, and on our skin. When Uğur and Özlem first started handling mRNA in Homburg, they had to go to extreme lengths to protect the vulnerable substance. A single beaker with an errant thumbprint on it would scupper an entire study. "We baked glassware at over three hundred degrees," Özlem says, "and developed specialized pipettes." Sebastian Kreiter, who later joined the couple's labs, recalls developing a certain amount of paranoia during their early experiments. "I would put my entire forearm in plastic bags and spray every surface," he says, using expensive RNAses-free water and specialized cleaning gear. "I lived in fear."

To make matters worse, mRNA was similarly unstable once it entered cells, where it was normally obliterated before cellular factories were able to produce a reasonable amount of protein. But while the rest of the world considered the fragility of mRNA an insurmountable obstacle, its degradation was seen as a "golden egg" by Uğur, Özlem, and the ragtag bunch of researchers who were independently committing themselves to the technology.

For a start, it meant the molecule would naturally disintegrate after fulfilling its function, making it much less likely to cause harm. More importantly, however, the evolutionary impulse that caused enzymes to eliminate mRNA was actually advantageous to those developing cancer therapies.

One of the things immunologists were discovering in the revolution of the 1990s was the dirty little secret that helped vaccines like Jenner's work. Since the early days of vaccine production, scientists had observed that doses that were combined with inactivated bacteria were more effective. Consequently, some developers deliberately added foreign substances like aluminum to vaccines to boost their potency. Toward the end of the twentieth century, it became clear why these methods were working.[17] Three researchers (Jules Hoffmann,[18] Bruce Beutler,[19] and Charles Janeway[20]) independently discovered that immune cells, such as DCs, were coated with specialized sensors that were triggered upon contact with certain substances commonly found on dangerous pathogens. It was not enough, they realized, for the patrolling generals to just collect intelligence; they needed to also be sufficiently panicked by the detection of a component on the invader to raise the alarm and rally the troops. Like a real general, they didn't commit all their forces to every fight—they assessed threats and made judgments based on DEFCON levels. The inactivated bacteria used in early vaccines was one crude way of alerting dendritic cells to a troublesome substance. But the best way of doing this was to add a well-defined adjuvant (from the Latin *adjuvare*, meaning "to help"), a substance that safely and directly triggered these newly discovered alarm buttons and helped to stimulate the immune system.[21]

One of the beauties of mRNA as a vaccine platform is that it acts as a *natural* adjuvant. The reason for this is simple. The oldest known threats to humankind were viruses made from RNA, just like the coronaviruses discovered in the twenty-first century. Some fifty thousand years ago, Neanderthals passed on their genetic defenses against RNA viruses to our ancestors,[22] and these sentries have kept guard at the portals of our anatomy ever since. Their singular mission is to stop RNA threats—which include menacing viruses, such as the flu, HIV, Zika, Ebola, and hepatitis C. This is why RNAses have evolved—to prevent foreign RNA from ever getting through the skin or into our bodies via our orifices.

The body's cells—which expect safe mRNA to come from their nucleus, not to suddenly be introduced from the outside—have developed further defenses against these intruders. Upon encountering foreign mRNA, their hardwired sensors trigger an alarm that sends troops scrambling to disarm the molecule. This so-called intrinsic adjuvant function would be enormously helpful to vaccine development, Uğur and Özlem believed. But while the promise was there, mRNA vaccines were still diamonds in the rough, and modulating their effectiveness was a struggle. Creating too much panic was not a desirable outcome; it could lead to severe side effects. The couple and their teams had to figure out how to ensure the immune troops were properly informed *and* stimulated by just the right amount. They needed to work on fine-tuning mRNA and on finding an effective way of delivering it to the right parts of the body.

A perfect example of the hurdles mRNA technology still had to overcome was exhibited by a study that Uğur and Özlem came across in their early research. Smita Nair, a postdoctoral researcher in the U.S., had been working on cell-based cancer vaccines. On one fateful day in 1995, her colleague (and future husband) David Boczkowski handed her a tube labeled "The Cure,"[23] containing mRNA extracted from a tumor cell. Rather than injecting the naked mRNA directly into the bloodstream, where it would struggle to survive, the duo introduced the mRNA into healthy dendritic cells extracted from mice and then administered these transfected cells back into the same rodents. Strong immune responses were induced, they explained in a paper published the following year, and consequently, the mice were protected against some cancers.[24] Eli Gilboa, the leader of Nair and Boczkowski's lab, was so excited by this discovery that he promptly started an mRNA company.

The key finding was a positive one—there was a way for mRNA therapies to elicit reasonable T-cell responses using dendritic cells. But the approach taken by Boczkowski, Nair and their team was cumbersome and expensive. If replicated as a real-world cancer drug, their method would entail drawing blood from a patient, cultivating and isolating healthy cells (a process that could take a couple of weeks), obtaining a sample of the tumor through biopsy (a couple of attempts could be needed to obtain sufficient material), extracting the RNA, and introducing it into healthy cells before administering the cells back to the patient. At every step, there was a high risk of contamination, and the process could only be done in well-equipped hospitals. The concept was beautiful, yet the technique was hardly more efficient than Jenner's. "The elegance and simplicity of mRNA was lost," says Uğur. "There had to be a simpler way."

By 1999, Uğur and Özlem's relentless quest for a simpler way led them to the Johannes Gutenberg University in Mainz, named after the city's most famous son, the inventor of the printing press. They had been invited to the university to establish an independent research group, funded by the German Research Foundation, and overseen by the Austrian oncologist Christoph Huber. In him, the couple found a kindred spirit. Christoph had been involved in trials of an early immunotherapy that tried to get the body to kill cancer cells by provoking a generalized immune response, but the drug failed, and participants suffered severe side effects to boot. Like Uğur and Özlem, he believed that the solution lay in making sure the immune system was activated in a very *specific* manner, and he created an environment enabling researchers to test their ideas to do just that.

Before moving to Mainz, however, Uğur took a year out to hone his skills at the renowned immunology department of the Universitätsspital in Zurich.[25] While Özlem recruited a research group, Uğur spent his weekdays in Switzerland, taking the train back to Germany on the weekends. The constant commuting was worth it. In Zurich, Uğur became friends with Thomas Kündig, a physician who had experimented with DNA vaccines and who had found that injecting them into the spleens of mice was superior to any other route in triggering an immune response. What Uğur learned was that the location to which a vaccine delivers its wanted poster really mattered.

The reason for this, the couple's team in Mainz later realized, was that not all dendritic cells, or generals, were created equal. The ones that resided in lymph nodes—of which the spleen is the largest—were particularly adept at capturing mRNA and making sure the instructions it carried were acted upon. These kidney bean–shaped organs, found under our armpits, in our groins, and at several other outposts in the body, are the information hubs of the immune system. They function as assembly points for our elite defenses—a biological Pentagon where intelligence gathered by dendritic cells is processed into instructions for the awaiting armies.

Further experiments revealed that dendritic cells in these Pentagons carried out their assignments with astonishing alacrity. While, as expected, the mRNA injected into lymph nodes was shredded by RNAses within minutes, the resident DCs worked quickly enough to suck up large amounts of it. They also produced large quantities of the proteins for which the molecules were encoded, to act as the wanted posters that warn the immune system's forces. DCs had evolved to be constantly scouting for foreign RNA, a feature that could now be exploited by immunologists. The specialized mechanism, coined *macropinocytosis*,[26] was later defined by the Mainz group.

Ironically, dendritic cells were the reason Uğur and Özlem had abandoned their first attempts at a DNA vaccine, when they found the cells did not ingest the molecule very well. When it came to mRNA, long dismissed as the "ugly stepchild" of DNA, DCs were not the barrier. They were the key to waking up the idle soldiers in the immune system's army bases.

Figuring out how the immune system worked, and what a vaccine would need to do to exploit it, was only half the battle. The other half was using these insights to improve mRNA, their favored platform, so that it could be translated into effective drugs for patients. Uğur and Özlem devoted the next couple of decades of their lives to tackling these tasks, in parallel.

Soon after their arrival in Mainz, word of the doctors' dual mission spread fast, and piqued the interest of scientists interested in similar topics. The first was Sebastian Kreiter. A trained physician, he had done his doctorate in the mid-1990s alongside Uğur and Özlem, at the Saarland University in Homburg, but had since lost touch with them. By chance, Sebastian ended up in Mainz too and was working under Christoph Huber, but he felt he was reaching a dead end in academia. He was about to give up and return to being a doctor on a hospital ward, but before he did so, he sought advice from the newly arrived Özlem, who was still furnishing the ninety square meters of space she and Uğur had been given to create a lab. Sitting on the only two chairs in this empty room, the pair talked for nearly an hour, Sebastian says, during which Özlem suggested several career options to her old friend. Then, at the end, she said, "But of course, you could also join *our* lab."

After taking some time off to get married, Sebastian entered that lab in the summer of 2001, expecting to work on viral vector drugs. It was on this basis that he had received the blessing of his superiors to abandon his existing research. But no sooner had he made himself comfortable than Uğur said, "Forget that. We are going to work on mRNA."

Two thousand kilometers away, Mustafa Diken was studying molecular biology and genetics in Ankara, Turkey. In the early 2000s, he spent his summer interning at a company in Istanbul, which was making use of one of Uğur and Özlem's earlier inventions: a technology called SEREX, which helped scientists discover tumor antigens. Intrigued by the innovative tool, Mustafa looked up the scientific papers behind it and couldn't help but notice the names of their authors. "I said, 'Oh, interesting, Turkish scientists in Germany!'" Mustafa says. "Then I just got their email addresses from the study and wrote to them." Hoping Uğur and Özlem would feel a sense of kinship, he asked to join their lab as a doctoral student. When he got no response, Mustafa persisted, until one day a message from Özlem landed in his inbox. She would soon be visiting family in Turkey, she said, and could allocate some time to talk to him.

The meeting, in a small, crowded café in the center of the Turkish capital, went well. Mustafa explained that he was interested in translational medicine, and his blend of determination and humility resonated with Özlem. She handed him a list of papers on mRNA, with which she suggested he familiarize himself. If it could be squared with the German authorities, she told him, he would be the perfect candidate to join their program in Mainz. A few months later, Mustafa found himself on a plane to Frankfurt, where he was greeted by a smiling Uğur, and spent his first night in the foreign country on the couple's couch.

Along with fifteen others, Sebastian and Mustafa formed the core of the closely knit team that, gently guided by Uğur and Özlem, bridged the gap between innovative science and pharmaceutical development. Quietly, they were refining the technologies that would become the mainstays of BioNTech's toolbox, a toolbox that was opened in early 2020, to take on COVID-19.

On a spring day in 2002, Uğur and Özlem took a brief break from bridging scientific gaps to tie the knot. There was no grand wedding plan or fancy venue booked. In fact, neither had given the details too much thought. A day before their nuptials, "they asked me and my colleague if we would come along as witnesses," says Helma Heinen, the couple's longtime personal assistant. Helma rushed out to buy some flowers and the next morning met her employers at the Mainz registry office. After a quick ceremony, the party of four headed back to work, and the newlyweds went straight to their lab. "That didn't seem unusual," says Helma. "It was always about the work."

When it came to that work, the first order of business was to profoundly improve the potency of the mRNA that made it to dendritic cells. This was particularly important for the couple's proposed cancer therapies, which had to induce an incredibly strong response if they were to successfully attack billions of tumor cells. The Mainz team therefore needed DCs to produce high amounts of the protein they encoded in synthetic mRNA—several wanted posters to plaster all over the immune system's barracks—and to do so for long enough for the immune system's sharp-shooters to be properly trained.

The problem, however, was that mRNA delivered from *outside* the body competes with mRNA already resident in host cells for time on the protein production line. Viruses and bacteria are dangerous because they often win this battle, using hostile methods. They invade a cell and block the translation of existing mRNA, to ensure their own replication. In principle, Uğur and Özlem believed they could get synthetic mRNA to learn from aggressive viruses. Or another strategy was to learn why some of the body's own mRNAs were particularly successful in producing large amounts of protein, while other, more average mRNAs in the body produced less. If the molecular messengers in the couple's drugs were similarly able to ensure that they were prioritized on cellular production lines, they would end up at the top of dendritic cells' to-do list and stay there for a while. In pursuit of this goal, the doctors and their newly formed core team transformed into a crack squad of biohackers.

All mRNA shares the same basic anatomy: a single strand containing up to several thousands of alternating sugar and phosphate groups. Attached to each sugar group is one of four bases, designated by the letters G, A, U, and C. The sequence of these letters determines the genetic information carried by the mRNA.

In the center of the mRNA strand is a larger coding segment marked by a universal start and stop sign, which contains the construction plan for the protein that the molecule compels cells to produce. The sections of the strand to the left and right of this coding region, the so-called backbone, are not translated into protein, but each of them has a specialized role. Together, they perform multiple functions, including ensuring that the strand is threaded into the cell's production factory in a readable manner, and that it remains on cellular assembly lines for long enough to make multiple copies of the encoded protein, rather than being pushed out of the way by existing cellular mRNAs.

The group focused on each of these components individually. For years, they systematically evaluated different optimizations, to see if they gave synthetic mRNA the equivalent of a VIP pass, so that their message was not ignored by the generals and was prioritized on protein production lines.

Their dedication paid off. One morning in December 2004, the team gathered around a flow cytometry machine—a device that looks like the loathed laser jet printers of old, but which counts and categorizes cells. Seventy-two hours earlier, Raouf Selmi, the team member with the steadiest hand, had carefully sliced open the armpit of a mouse using a scalpel the size of a nail file, exposing its tiny lymph node. After posing for a picture to mark this historic moment, he injected some optimized mRNA with pinpoint accuracy. Now, the do-or-die results were coming up on a computer screen. Not only had the mRNA been taken up by dendritic cells, but the octopus-like creatures had expressed enough of the protein for which the mRNA had been coded to prompt a mass deployment of the immune system's sharpshooters. The scan showed a blue mass, the lymph node, covered with millions of purple dots, as if it had broken out in a severe rash. The flecks represented the specialized weapons that Uğur and Özlem had spent decades trying to coax into action: T-cells. The biohackers had successfully manipulated their targets. A new generation of cancer drugs based on an underestimated molecule suddenly seemed viable.

By 2006, having combined several tweaks into one mRNA backbone, the couple and their team achieved a five-thousand-fold increase in the immune response prompted by a strand of mRNA. Uğur presented the data of this breakthrough in a nationwide competition organized by the German ministry of research, emerging as one of the winners. His prize was €6 million of funding, awarded on the condition that it be used to found a company within two years. The foundation stone for BioNTech had been laid.

Thousands of miles away, another dogged biohacker was working on her own solution to mRNA's drawbacks.

Katalin Karikó had first learned about the molecule in 1976 from a university lecturer in Szeged, a city in the south of her native Hungary. Intrigued, she immediately decided to pursue a doctorate in the subject and set about doing experiments in the institution's cigarette-smoke-filled labs. Her research helped her flee the then communist country, after she received an offer to further her research at Temple University in Pennsylvania. As the regime would not allow her to export foreign currency worth more than $50, she sold the family car for $900 and, along with her husband's allowance, stuffed the equivalent of $1,000 in their daughter's teddy bear,[27] before heading to the United States.

The next two decades, however, provided a relentless series of setbacks. When Katalin tried to inject mRNA strands into mice, some of the rodents died, she says, possibly because of the inflammation caused by the immune response to enormous doses. Plus, the biochemist was running into similar problems to Uğur and Özlem, in that not enough of the mRNA's instructions were being translated by cells. Eventually, the University of Pennsylvania, to which Katalin had since moved, grew tired of funding her pet project and forced her to choose between a demotion or moving to a new area of research.

Katalin, who chose the former, was soon to find luck, however, in the form of Drew Weissman, an immunologist who had arrived in Philadelphia after working at the National Institutes of Health with none other than Anthony Fauci. In 1998, they met while jostling over a photocopy machine, which was in high demand in the age before scientific journals could be easily found online, and the two got chatting about her mRNA frustrations. Together, they found a way to make the molecule stable enough to ensure it prompted robust protein production when introduced into cells.

The duo realized that by substituting the U (which stands for *uridine*) in the mRNA code with a naturally occurring alternative, such as methylpseudouridine, the molecule would effectively be placed in "stealth mode." It would not be properly detected by the immune system's innate receptors, the ones that have evolved to react to foreign mRNA. It would slip through largely unnoticed.

Despite this breakthrough, which was patented in 2006, Katalin continued to suffer professional indignities. In 2013, when she returned from a conference in Japan, she found her chair in the hallway and her office cleared to make way for another researcher. Later the same year, in Europe to attend a tournament in which her daughter, an Olympic rower, was competing, Katalin traveled to BioNTech to meet Uğur. She had already visited CureVac, which had shown an interest in her innovations, and she was relieved to find herself in the company of fellow mRNA enthusiasts. It was the "first time in my life that I didn't have to explain that RNA is good, because all of the people who were there were believers," she says. But she was even more enamored by her reception in Mainz. She talked with Uğur for hours, comparing notes on their common passion, before he asked her to join the business. A few months later, BioNTech announced that she was joining the team as a vice president. "My chairman laughed at me," Katalin remembers. "He said: 'The company doesn't even have a website!'"

BioNTech was indeed keeping a low profile, but Uğur and Özlem's teams had not been idle. In 2012, the Mainz group moved from experiments with mice to testing their constructs on humans. After getting the go-ahead from the German regulator, they injected naked uridine mRNA into the lymph nodes in the groins of patients with advanced melanoma. The process was not straightforward; doctors had to use ultrasound machines and jelly, of the type often used for baby scans, to ensure the needle reached all the way into the bean-shaped organ. The results, however, were worth the fuss. Dozens of patients mounted robust T-cell responses against the encoded cancer antigens. "We proved that if you inject a little bit of mRNA into one stupid lymph node, the body does the rest of the work," says Sebastian Kreiter. It was now clear that human dendritic cells, especially those in the body's Pentagons, eagerly engulfed mRNA and acted upon its instructions.

The mechanism might have been clear, but the mode of administration—into the groin—was less than ideal. Besides, Uğur had wondered, given that injecting into two lymph nodes at the top of the legs had such a strong effect, "how substantial could the immune response be if a vaccine got into all lymphatic tissues around the body and recruited *all* the resident DCs into action?"

Into the lab Uğur, Özlem, and the team went. Intravenous injection, they knew, was the most efficient way to get the widest and most systemic distribution of a drug within the body. However, due to the presence of the RNA-zapping forces, mRNA would need some protection on its journey through the bloodstream to the lymph nodes. There were a host of fancy technologies that could be used to achieve this, but the group opted for the simplest—lipid formulations. One of these formulations, containing microscopic globules of fat, would years later become a crucial part of BioNTech's coronavirus vaccine plans. Lipids would protect the mRNA from patrolling enzymes and prevent the molecule from getting stuck in the liver or the lungs along the way to its destinations.

Back in the 2010s, the doctors and their team cycled through dozens of lipids, all with slightly altered chemical makeups, to find the perfect match for their mRNA platforms. "At the beginning, it was purely trial and error," says Özlem, "but then we started to learn." The group began to understand that it was not only the lipids that mattered but the proportions in which they were combined with mRNA. After performing hundreds of experiments, they found that nanoparticles of a specific size and with a well-defined mRNA-to-lipid ratio did the trick.

The message encoded in the mRNA and sent through the bloodstream reached the generals in the Pentagons of the body, who were sufficiently alerted by its contents to train their troops. The immune response from vaccines containing the Mainz's group's biohacked mRNA backbone components encased with these lipids was excellent. Wanted posters were plastered over the immune enforcers' barracks.

Uğur and Özlem, sensing they were close to their original goal of creating potent mRNA cancer vaccines that could be injected intravenously, accelerated their discoveries into the clinic. In 2014, BioNTech started a new clinical trial and treated the first patient with this newly invented lipid-encapsulated mRNA vaccine.[28] Their breakthrough was published in a landmark paper in the prestigious journal *Nature*.[29] A few years later, in 2017, Uğur was confident enough to tell *Nature* that he was "absolutely convinced" mRNA technology was the future. In contrast to the disappointment of DNA vaccines, mRNA was "not hype," he told the writer. "It remained under the radar for many years, and it's now mature enough to fulfill promises."[30]

In October 2018, Uğur followed up on the 2014 trial in which the intravenous mRNA had been administered. He presented the data from several dozen melanoma patients treated in this study to immunologists gathered in a ballroom on the eighth floor of the New York Marriott Marquis[31] in Times Square, for an event entitled "Translating Science into Survival." A day earlier, James P. Allison—a cancer immunologist, who along with Tasuku Honjo had just been awarded the Nobel Prize in Medicine for marshaling the body's existing defenses to fight advanced tumors[32]—had appeared at the conference and received a rapturous reception. The crowd was convinced that they were finally entering the era of cancer immunotherapy, and Uğur gave them even more to cheer about. While Özlem watched on in the audience, he told them that after receiving BioNTech's mRNA drug, several patients' tumors had shrunk. All had developed strong T-cell responses,[33] and in some cases, billions of these sharpshooters had been deployed. The emperor of all maladies was finally faced with a powerful adversary: all the weapons in the immune system's arsenal had been trained, with laser-like focus, on this dreadful disease.

Here, after more than two hundred years of vaccinology, was the prospect of an efficient system that could finally replace Jenner's rudimentary technique. As long as optimized mRNA was delivered to the lymphoid tissue in a suitable wrapper, dendritic cells—the generals—idling about in those organs would pick it up and raise the alarm at a sufficient pitch to prompt a powerful immune response.

Little did the couple know, however, that the technology they were on the cusp of perfecting would be catapulted onto a much larger stage in just fifteen months' time and that its potential to end a pandemic would have the rest of humanity holding its breath.

THE TESTS

COVID-19 is an infectious disease, but in January 2020, BioNTech was still chiefly a cancer company. It's not that Uğur and Özlem, who had initially bonded over a shared desire to defeat one of humankind's most intractable enemies, weren't interested in viruses. They had always known that the armada of technologies they were developing to target tumors could be used to improve vaccines and treatments for other maladies. The couple's initial business model for their first firm, Ganymed, included a technology invented by Uğur that could quickly identify the genetic sequence of a new pathogen and develop antibodies against it. "Already back then," says Özlem, "epidemics and pandemics were close to our hearts."

Since there was no medical application for the invention of commercial interest to investors, Ganymed focused exclusively on cancer instead. Later, at BioNTech, when Uğur and Özlem had more leeway, they revisited the idea of applying their innovations to infectious disease vaccines. From an immunological perspective, such products were easier to develop than cancer drugs. But the market for infectious disease vaccines was controlled by a few large, and conservative, companies who would view the couple's novel technologies with suspicion. Going it alone was not an option either. The development of such vaccines required much larger Phase 3 trials than cancer therapies, involving tens of thousands of subjects and a global distribution and commercialization network. Huge investments and the hiring of thousands of employees would be required, and BioNTech was a small spin-off from a university in Mainz.

Uğur and Özlem decided to focus on the long term. They were content to let others pick the low-hanging fruit of vaccines against common infectious diseases for which drugs, however imperfect, already existed. "We wanted to focus on our strengths," says Uğur, "on diseases such as the 'big three'—HIV, tuberculosis, and malaria—that are so complex or difficult to treat that they cannot be adequately addressed with conventional technologies."

First, though, the couple had to pick a lower-hanging fruit to lay the groundwork for an infectious diseases unit. Together with their team, they chose to focus first on influenza—a well-known virus that had been studied for decades. Because plenty of flu vaccines already existed, it would also be easy to judge how well drugs based on the technologies in BioNTech's steadily growing mRNA toolbox really worked, by comparing them with conventional shots. In 2011, the company secured German government grants for this pilot program, which Uğur and Özlem deliberately kept out of sight.

The first employee with specific infectious-disease know-how was hired two years later. At first, Stephanie Erbar found she was not central to BioNTech's operations. "People were afraid of being infected," she says of her cancer colleagues. "I was only allowed to work in the labs in the afternoons or evenings, when no one else was there." Her first office was in the Tote Taube, or "dead pigeon" room, so named because of a deceased bird that was stuck on the skylight, slowly rotting away.

Things brightened up in 2014, when BioNTech employed its second virologist, a young animal disease expert named Annette Vogel. A south German native, she had studied in Tübingen before joining a federal research institute based in the medieval city. After a few years on the job, her employer relocated to Riems, a small peninsula in the Baltic Sea, populated almost exclusively by infectious disease specialists and their test subjects: a few dozen sheep and cows. Annette found the isolation too much to bear and was about to quit when she heard from a friend who had worked for BioNTech. The company was looking for people with just her skills, she was told, but when Annette looked online for a job description, she began to wonder if she was the subject of a practical joke. Her search returned no meaningful results. It was 2014, and BioNTech, which in just six years' time would develop one of the most important drugs in the history of medicine, still did not have a website.

Nonetheless, after a call with Özlem and a visit to Mainz, Annette agreed to join the infectious diseases "team." Together with Stephanie, she started to cautiously adapt BioNTech's cancer technologies for use against viruses, enlisting the help of academic institutions who understood the characteristics of particular pathogens. To Annette, who was perhaps unaware of the foundation laid by her cancer vaccine colleagues, it seemed like virology "was still largely a hobby for BioNTech."

In 2015, after a technician was hired, the infectious diseases duo became a trio and began to work on their first serious project—a European initiative led by Imperial College London to develop protective and therapeutic HIV vaccines. Then came collaborations with Bayer's animal health division on vaccines for farm animals and with the University of Pennsylvania on a plethora of pathogens.[1] The Gates Foundation invested soon thereafter, and a fully fledged influenza project with Pfizer followed in 2018. But while fellow mRNA companies Moderna and CureVac were moving their infectious disease vaccines into the clinic, similar programs at BioNTech, which was still prioritizing cancer projects, remained in the exploratory phase.

When COVID-19 struck China, the closest the company had come to a human trial for an infectious disease vaccine was via a loose alliance with Imperial's lead immunologist, Robin Shattock. A UK-funded vaccine against Ebola, the Marburg virus, and Lassa fever, had been registered for a Phase 1 study with the British regulator, MHRA, but was still months away from going ahead. This project, and those like it, were barely mentioned in BioNTech's public presentations. In Uğur's speech at the J. P. Morgan conference in San Francisco at the start of 2020, BioNTech's infectious disease pipeline was first mentioned at the bottom of slide number forty-two. The company was still, in the eyes of the biotechnology world, concentrating on cancer. Beneath the surface there were, of course, hundreds of people in Mainz whose work would feed into the development of vaccines against viruses. But when Uğur launched

Project Lightspeed, the unit *explicitly* dedicated to infectious diseases, now run by Annette, consisted of just fifteen people.

Scientifically speaking, this was not much of an obstacle. Yes, most of the work done by Uğur and Özlem over the decades, diving into the depths of immunotherapy, was done with cancer in mind. But as this work was "about redirecting the immune system's natural mechanisms, which were developed to fend off viruses," Özlem explains, "it was actually a small step from taking all this knowledge and using it for its original purpose—namely, protection from viruses."

BioNTech had amassed quite some knowledge. It had quietly developed four versions of synthetic mRNA, with individual building blocks removed, replaced, or reconfigured to augment the molecule's natural powers. The first and most extensively vetted one, uridine mRNA, or uRNA, had the ability to provoke particularly strong T-cell responses by virtue of its adjuvant—or alarm signaling—activity. When wrapped in the lipid BioNTech had built for intravenous injection, it had triggered such responses in cancer patients at very low doses. But the uRNA had not yet been combined with intramuscular lipids—the ones needed for a COVID-19 shot. Because these contain their own supplementary adjuvant, a vaccine containing the lipids *and* uRNA could prove too powerful, causing flu-like symptoms.

The second format was modified mRNA, or modRNA. This platform included, on top of the improvements made by the couple, the discovery patented by Katalin Karikó and Drew Weissman, who had substituted one of the four letters of the molecule's code, putting it in a stealth mode. The duo's breakthrough had been licensed by BioNTech,[2] and it helped modRNA be well tolerated by humans, causing few side effects. However, the modifications to modRNA strongly blunted the *intrinsic* adjuvant ability of the molecule to panic the patrolling generals of the immune system into action, when introduced from outside the body. In contrast to the uRNA, the modRNA needed the help of intramuscular lipids, with their adjuvant effect, to compensate, and it was unclear whether the fatty globules would make up the shortfall.

Self-amplifying mRNA, or saRNA, and trans-amplifying mRNA, or taRNA,[3] were more recent arrivals in the BioNTech lineup—rookies with enormous potential. As their names suggest, they come with their own "copy machine," or ability to replicate, dramatically increasing and prolonging the production of a vaccine antigen, such as the coronavirus spike protein, on cellular manufacturing lines. But these were new platforms and had never been tested in humans at all, with or without lipids. It was not known whether the vaccine potency observed in mice injected with formulations based on saRNA and taRNA could be reproduced in humans.

Long before the coronavirus came along, these platforms were continuously being improved upon by an interdisciplinary group Uğur had formed in 2013, dubbed the Optimal mRNA Team.[4] In bimonthly meetings, the latest data from experiments with the different technologies were discussed in detail and challenged with scientific rigor. Hypotheses were put forward to be subsequently buried or confirmed. Sometimes, the jovial gatherings felt like a university debating club. All participants, whatever their level of experience, were encouraged to adopt contrary positions and refine their arguments, fueled by coffee and cookies. Bets were placed on what the results of planned investigations would be. Not only did these discussions lead to numerous refinements to the parts of the mRNA backbone that can be tweaked to make vaccines more potent, but they also led to improved manufacturing and purification methods, which generated higher yields and improved mRNA activity. Each of the team's discoveries were layered upon previous breakthroughs. "You can't ever reach perfection," says Uğur. "The optimal version was always only temporarily the optimal version."

These improvements were still ongoing in February 2020, and the Lightspeed experts did not want to bet on a single mRNA format without having some clinical data to go on. But their reticence to pick just one of the innovations in BioNTech's toolbox for a COVID-19 vaccine was not merely down to a desire to test the relative merits of individual mRNA platforms. It was also due to a lack of evidence for how these technologies would work when combined with certain lipids. Years earlier, when optimizing their cancer vaccines, Uğur and Özlem had discovered that these wrappers led to a "multiplication of mRNA's impact." Not only could the composition of these fatty globules be tweaked to enable intravenous or intramuscular administration of mRNA, but it could also regulate the molecule's precise destination, allowing vaccine developers to choose the organs and cell types to which they wanted their cargo delivered. How the lipid chosen for Project Lightspeed would behave in combination with each of the company's mRNA platforms remained an open question.

Since the couple first learned the art of lipid nanoparticle formulation (to enable them to inject cancer vaccines directly into the bloodstream of cancer patients, rather than lymph nodes in the groin), they and their team had climbed a steep learning curve. An ever-expanding specialist group at BioNTech continued to systematically test cocktails of various lipids, for various purposes, one of which was to enable the vaccines to be injected directly into human muscle.

The mission of these new lipids was the same as those developed for cancer vaccines: to get mRNA to dendritic cells, or generals, sitting in the body's largest lymph nodes, or Pentagons. Sticking with their open-minded approach, BioNTech's teams, although masters of molecular disguise themselves, tested their own lipid compositions alongside those created by other, more specialist companies. Among the best ones they identified were formulations made by the Canadian company Acuitas.

For use in humans, all drug components have to be produced in a replicable and quality-controlled manner. When it comes to lipid nanoparticle formulations, this process is particularly challenging and takes a year to set up. Prior to the fateful weekend in January 2020, when Uğur and Özlem decided to develop a coronavirus vaccine, there was no hurry within BioNTech to make drugs given via intramuscular injection. There was only one intramuscular lipid that could be manufactured at a moment's notice: an Acuitas formulation originally destined to be tested in BioNTech's flu vaccine partnership with Pfizer.

It was this lipid that the couple and their team had presented to the German regulator in that first meeting in February. But while they knew the formulation was safe, they did not know whether it would render the mRNA platforms they had worked on for years more effective or less. Moderna and CureVac, who had both launched coronavirus vaccine projects, had plenty of clinical data on the mRNA formats and lipid formulations they intended to use. BioNTech had none.

For yet another reason, the company seemed among the least likely candidates to develop a COVID-19 vaccine at all, never mind to do so to Uğur's timeline: the end of 2020. There was a full lap of the track between BioNTech and its competitors. To catch up, the Lightspeed team needed to identify a winning construct, and fast. There was no time for iterative improvements, for pursuing perfection. They would have to test at least twenty possible permutations of a COVID-19 vaccine, in different doses, in parallel. Vaccines based on modRNA, uRNA, saRNA, and taRNA, wrapped in Acuitas's lipids and coding for slightly different versions of the full spike protein or the receptor-binding domain, would each be evaluated, *simultaneously*.

Technicians would work around the clock to see how successfully each vaccine summoned the combined forces of the immune system—the sharpshooting T-cells and antibodies—and how long this effect lasted. Meanwhile, on the same floor, specialist teams would design experiments to test whether the constructs were safe in mammals. To save time later on, materials would be produced, from day one, to the high standard required for clinical trials.

All the scientific and entrepreneurial expertise Uğur and Özlem had gained since locking eyes on a cancer ward would be thrown at this disease. Their team would, by process of elimination, identify the candidate that could be delivered to billions of people worldwide. First, however, there was the small matter of producing test batches of vaccine.

Like every other vaccine-maker, BioNTech had been given a helping hand when the genetic code of the coronavirus—sequenced thanks to the quick thinking of Zhang Yongzhen, a professor at the Shanghai Public Health Clinical Center—was uploaded on January 11, 2020, onto the open-source website Virological. Uğur had studied this molecular blueprint on that fateful weekend at the end of the month and had used it to sketch blueprints for several vaccine candidates. But these were just formulas on paper or, more accurately, on-screen.

The first step to making actual vaccine material was to create DNA hard copies for the candidates, which would then be used as a template to make RNA. Stephanie Hein, the molecular biologist in charge of stocking BioNTech's RNA warehouse—a physical repository of antigens, or targets, for the company's vaccines and therapies—worked fast to map out the genetic sequences for these templates. They contained up to four thousand nucleotides and had to be assembled from between fifty to eighty smaller building blocks as a perfect, error-free code consisting of the nucleotides G, A, T, and C. Once complete, the sequences were to be cloned and checked for accuracy.

The laboratory procedures for this approach, known as *gene synthesis*, had been established at BioNTech years earlier and were, by now, routine. However, cloning the DNA template for some candidates proved, unexpectedly, to be a tortuous task. Try as they might, Stephanie and her team could not combine individual nucleotides in the right order or fuse segments correctly. They explored every possible solution, but each time they analyzed cloned templates, something in the sequence was off.

Another team was already eagerly waiting to receive the DNA so that they could prepare the production of actual vaccine candidates, and the delay threatened to push back Uğur's ambitious schedule. Much greater challenges lay ahead, but in mid-February, the Lightspeed team was in danger of stumbling over what should have been the smallest of hurdles.

Reminiscing about this unanticipated challenge, Uğur is philosophical. "Sometimes," he muses, "a lab feels like it's jinxed. Out of the blue, tried-and-tested daily procedures cease to work, and errors creep in. You start troubleshooting. You doubt everything. You change reagents, repeat every step, and still, everything fails. You feel like a football team that is unable to complete simple passes, because the ball keeps bouncing away. It gnaws at your self-confidence. In these situations, you can't put pressure on a team. You can't criticize them; you have to encourage them and build up their self-belief. And then, all of a sudden, the ball starts rolling again, and everyone plays like world champions."

At first, that sudden switch seemed elusive. In fact, Stephanie suffered a further setback when one of her colleagues became pregnant. As kanamycin, an antibiotic used in the cloning process, can be toxic to a fetus, she was immediately banished from the lab. "We went from three team members to two, and one of them was part-time," says Stephanie, who had no choice but to don her lab coat for the first time in two years and do some pipetting herself.

Then, one day in February, two biochemists—Thomas Ziegenhals and Johanna Drögemüller—came up with an ingenious work-around. Instead of waiting for the synthesis to be successful, they suggested that manufacturing teams start planning their processes using existing DNA templates from BioNTech's RNA warehouse. These templates had comparable features and were of a similar length to those needed for the coronavirus vaccines. The move took some pressure off Stephanie and her gene synthesis team, who could now focus on correcting errors, knowing that they were not holding up the entire project. And with that, just as abruptly as the cloning problems had appeared, they disappeared. The new sequences that came in turned out to be correct. Stephanie's team began to create one perfect clone after another. Construction of the first vaccine was completed in late February.

On March 2, the first batch of RNA, using Stephanie's successful DNA template, was produced by the manufacturing experts who had prepared for this stage with Thomas and Johanna's warehouse solution. The material was poured into a 50 milliliter bag and immediately deep-frozen at minus 70 degrees Celsius as a precaution to ensure the molecules' stability. Outside BioNTech's Mainz HQ, a car was waiting to drive it—at great expense—to Polymun, the family business in Vienna with whom BioNTech had developed a relationship and which had the expertise to combine the mRNA with Acuitas's lipids. A couple of days later, a small Styrofoam box containing frozen vials full of vaccine would be driven back over the border to BioNTech. With each of the twenty constructs, the trip would be repeated. Emails would go back and forth with constant updates in the style of Secret Service agents chaperoning a president. "The RNA has left the building," they would read, or simply: "On the move."

The ball had started rolling again, and the team was playing like champions.

With the first vials soon to arrive back at the Mainz campus, a team led by Annette Vogel began designing a vaccine beauty contest to pit the twenty candidates against one another. The goal was to determine which of the contestants induced immune responses at particularly low doses—a measure the Lightspeed team would use to choose the constructs for further clinical testing. These criteria would also inform the decision, in a few months' time, as to which vaccine BioNTech would enter in a Phase 3 study and eventually provide to the world.

The first, and simplest, test the team planned to carry out was in vitro: literally in a glass dish. Two technicians would transfect cells with the mRNA and wait to see if they produced perfect replicas of the coronavirus spike protein. While scientifically unspectacular, such tests would later be crucial for checking the quality of the vaccine batches produced for clinical or commercial use.

Next came animal studies, carried out at a separate location. For these, the vaccine candidates would be administered to groups of eight rodents, in three different dosages: low, medium, and high. Once the mice were all dosed and monitored for signs of side effects, their blood would be taken at several intervals over six weeks to run hundreds of make-or-break tests.

A group led by Lena Kranz and Mathias Vormehr would use the samples to look for both kinds of T-cells: CD4s, also known as *helper cells*, the initiators and orchestrators of the immune response, and patrolling CD8s, with their innate "x-ray vision" that allows them to identify and kill camouflaged enemies. The Mulder and Scully of BioNTech (the duo often conclude each other's sentences), Lena and Mathias contributed to the development of the company's mRNA cancer vaccines as graduate students and had since become world-leading T-cell detectives. They would be able to tell whether T-cells reacted to the coronavirus spike protein as expressed by vaccine candidates and if they carried out the *desired* immune response or one that could make COVID-19 worse for those infected. But Lena and Mathias's tests were complex and would take a while to complete.

Meanwhile, to find out if the vaccine constructs were inducing enough antibodies in mice, Annette's team would use a well-established technique using enzyme-linked immunosorbent assays, fondly anthropomorphized in the trade by the acronym ELISA.

Similar to the tests that would become commonplace later on in the pandemic to detect asymptomatic spread of COVID-19, and to ascertain whether recovered patients had antibodies, the ELISA was relatively simple. But it could not differentiate between antibodies that merely bind to the virus and those that bind in a manner that *neutralizes* the threat, stopping it from entering healthy cells. To find out whether antibodies were doing the trick, Annette's team needed to develop a gold standard experiment, known as a *virus neutralization test,* or VNT.

BioNTech had the *technical* capabilities to measure for neutralizing antibodies. The company had performed such tests in the early stages of its collaboration with Pfizer on a flu vaccine. Its teams would cultivate the virus and add it to healthy cells, together with serum containing potentially neutralizing antibodies. After five days, they would check to see if the cells had died—or whether infection had been prevented. All of this was done on-site in BioNTech's labs—the handling of influenza was subject to only minor compliance restrictions. But regulators required more safeguards for handling a new, highly infectious virus, which had, by the end of February 2020, claimed the lives of three thousand people worldwide.[5]

Since the 1970s, a series of safety measures had been introduced for working with dangerous microorganisms, and a tiering system was established. Experiments with Ebola—which, with a mortality rate of roughly 90 percent, was categorized as one of the most hazardous pathogens—had to take place in specialized biosafety-level (BSL) 4 laboratories. Those who handled it were required to wear full-body hazmat suits—of the sort seen in disaster movies—and breathe through their own air supply. Influenza, which has been around for centuries, and for which most humans now have some natural defenses, was categorized as BSL-2 in the jargon, meaning that those working with it must take standard precautions, such as wearing gloves and a mask, but need little in terms of specialist equipment. Live samples of the COVID-19 virus landed somewhere in between, at BSL-3. This meant it could only be handled in a biosafety cabinet, a work space protected by a glass screen, with a small gap through which technicians can insert their arms. The lab itself would need to have gas-impermeable walls, ceilings, and floors; an anteroom with sealable doors; and be designed to withstand earthquakes. The airflow would have to be closely controlled and all fixtures able to withstand regular cleaning with industrial-strength chemicals.[6]

BioNTech had no BSL-3 labs. The tests for neutralizing antibodies would have to be done externally using a contractor. Not only would this be extremely costly, as thousands of samples needed to be sent back and forth in deep-frozen containers, but it would also slow things down. The company would no doubt operate only during regular working hours and test the constructs sequentially, rather than in parallel. The Lightspeed team would get their first glimpse at the data in three or four weeks' time, once it had all been gathered, formulated, and double-checked for errors. The assessment of the vaccines would be slowed considerably.

But there was an even bigger problem. The external vendor most capable of testing for neutralizing antibodies at short notice was, as luck would have it, based in the heart of Italy's Tuscany region, which was fast becoming a COVID-19 hot spot. The north of the country was already in partial lockdown, and the virus had already been identified in all of Italy's twenty regions. Even if the contractor's lab was able to remain operational and staff weren't infected en masse, shipments of mice serum samples to and from the area were likely to be greatly disrupted. BioNTech needed an alternative, and fast. Miraculously, a solution emerged from the most unlikely of places.

Alex Muik, a locally educated biochemist, was not on the Lightspeed team. He had first heard about the project from colleagues attending other departmental meetings and, over discussions at the watercooler, had learned of the trouble that Annette's unit was encountering in getting the testing process up and running. Although he was busy enough working on one of the company's cancer drugs, this new information shone out like a Bat-Signal to Alex. Years earlier, in the first stretch of his scientific career, he had gained specific skills that were of limited use to his current employer. Now, however, his expertise would come into play.

In the decade before he moved to Mainz, Alex had worked with oncolytic viruses—specific pathogens that were particularly efficient at entering tumor cells and ripping them apart—in pursuit of an early version of immunotherapy.[7] One such pathogen was the vesicular stomatitis virus, or VSV, a less dangerous relation of rabies that causes flu-like symptoms in humans. As a Ph.D. student, Alex had worked on tweaking the VSV, which harmed the nervous system, to make it safe for administration to cancer patients. He did this by splicing in harmless proteins from other viruses and found that VSV was amenable to being mucked around with. The process was like removing bricks from a Jenga tower; the parts of the virus that caused severe disease could be carefully replaced, without causing the entire construct to fall apart. Alex managed to reduce the toxicity of VSV by a factor of one million.

In 2016, keen to work on innovations that could be brought into the clinic, he applied for a job at BioNTech and was hired. Thrilled as he was to join an ambitious start-up, Alex knew he would be leaving much of his previous expertise behind. At BioNTech, he would not be working on oncolytic viruses but rather on an immunotherapy for improving T-cell responses against cancer. Then came COVID-19.

On March 2, after hearing of Project Lightspeed's testing woes, Alex sent an email to Annette, politely inquiring how she planned to test for neutralizing antibodies. In the exchange that followed, he learned about the plan that involved using an Italian company soon to be engulfed by coronavirus cases. The alternative—setting up an in-house BSL-3 lab with all the specialist equipment required—would take too long. But Alex had a proposal: "I can develop an in-house test."

Instead of using a live sample of the coronavirus, he said, the company could call upon his old friend—the vesicular stomatitis virus. In his earlier career, Alex had replaced the dangerous bricks in the Jenga tower of VSV with harmless proteins. This time, he could replace the harmful elements with the isolated spike protein from SARS-CoV-2, which would be integrated into the virus's genetic envelope and stripped of its ability to infect. This would create a *pseudo*virus, which contained the part of the coronavirus that BioNTech was hoping to target with its vaccines, but was unable to cause COVID-19. Alex's construct would be nothing more than a harmless impersonator.

To see if antibodies deployed by BioNTech's vaccine constructs were accurate and strong enough to beat back COVID-19, the Lightspeed team would be able to observe whether they were able to deactivate the spike protein, perfectly replicated using a VSV wrapper. Most importantly, the VSV pseudovirus would be classified as a BSL-1 substance, meaning it could be handled in BioNTech's existing labs. "Just an idea," Alex wrote to Annette. "What do you think?"

Such tests, Annette knew, were frequently used to give scientists an early indication of whether neutralizing antibodies were in play. BioNTech, however, had never needed to use the method before, and it would be a challenge to set up a pseudovirus test from scratch, at a high enough standard to support real-world drug development, rather than research. Specialized equipment needed to be identified and ordered, reagents needed to be purchased, and all the elements calibrated to assure consistent results. But Alex was confident. Leaning on his previous experience, he told Annette he could get the test up and running, and fast. "That would be really amazing," she replied. "But I'm really swamped. We don't have the capacity to back you up."

Undeterred, Alex plowed ahead. First, however, he needed to get hold of the VSV, the virus in whose company he had spent most of his days as a young scientist. Specifically, he needed a plasmid—a molecule containing a fraction of DNA that contains the code for the pathogen. BioNTech, which did not work with VSV, had no such material in storage, so Alex called up some old friends. "I need some VSV plasmids, and I need them now," he pleaded. Days later, he loaded a dry-ice container onto the back seat of his white VW Golf to retrieve his emergency order.

One key ingredient, however, was still missing. To get the modified VSV to express the spike protein, he needed to get hold of the genetic material of the protrusion in its original form—not the stabilized version Stephanie and her team had struggled to produce in-house. Unbeknownst to Alex, his boss was already several steps ahead. On February 21, Uğur had emailed project manager Corinna Rosenbaum to say that Sino Biological, a Chinese company with a campus west of Frankfurt, was offering to supply its customers with the DNA template encoding for the full sequence of the coronavirus spike protein. Corinna, who was dropping her son off at his kindergarten, immediately called the company to get more details. She then bought two coffees and headed over to BioNTech, where she waited outside Stephanie's office, keen to check with her if the product matched the Lightspeed team's testing needs. It did, but since the DNA template was synthesized in China, she learned, it would take weeks to arrive. Corinna conveyed these concerns to Uğur, who replied, "I know, and I have ordered it already with my private credit card."

On March 5, as Alex was gathering instruments and materials for his inventive test, he received a message from Uğur. The good news was that a test tube containing the DNA encoding for the spike protein had arrived in Mainz. The bad news was that Sino Biological had delivered the parcel to the receptionist at TRON, a research institute Uğur had founded ten years earlier with Özlem and their mentor, Christoph Huber, which was based just down the road. On Sierk Poetting's instructions, the Lightspeed team were keeping their contact with outsiders to a minimum to avoid infection. Fetching the test tube in person seemed risky, so Alex arranged to meet a TRON staffer outside, opposite BioNTech's HQ. A few minutes later, in what must have looked like a drug deal to passersby, two masked men walked up to a bus shelter, and the swap was made.

While Alex worked on replicating the precious DNA template—the first fragment of the actual coronavirus to enter BioNTech's campus—Annette and her team received the first batch of lipid-encapsulated mRNA back from Vienna. On March 9, having driven overnight from Polymun, a black car pulled up outside the headquarters with a few dozen vials containing just enough material for initial animal studies. By March 11, the vaccines were being injected into mice. On the same day, the World Health Organization declared a pandemic.

Events began to escalate quickly. On March 13, the majority of Germany's states ordered an immediate shutdown of schools and nurseries. Rhineland-Palatinate, of which Mainz is the capital, was not among them, but Sierk soon had a staffing problem on his hands nonetheless, thanks to the country's federal system. Many of the Lightspeed team were commuting from the neighboring states of Baden-Württemberg and Hesse, where only children of key workers could be dropped off at kindergartens. Authorities in those states had never even heard of BioNTech, never mind its vaccine program, and were refusing to look after employees' kids. An emergency crèche was set up in the boardroom on the company's main campus, while Sierk's team navigated local bureaucracies to obtain a letter stating that BioNTech was crucial to the fight against coronavirus.

A similar problem prevented the team from obtaining enough personal protective equipment. Gloves and gowns were in short supply and reserved for institutions considered *system relevant*. BioNTech lacked such a status, so lab manager François Perrineau and Jasmina Alatovic, the company's comms chief, began calling politicians, explaining the work that was being done and asking what the company needed to do to be prioritized for the purchase of safety products. An acute shortage of disposable aprons and the like was already hampering the Lightspeed team's record-breaking efforts. China's Fosun even sent face masks over to help their new partner. "At one point, we had to reuse gloves," says François. "It was awful."

Germany's borders to Austria, France, and Switzerland were also being closed, and curfews were introduced in areas with high infection rates. Angela Merkel had so far stopped short of imposing a national lockdown, but Sierk, who was out buying pizza for his now homeschooled children when the news of increasing restrictions trickled through, saw the writing on the wall. The first coronavirus death in Germany had been confirmed days earlier, and the number of fatalities had rapidly increased to eight.[8] Just six weeks after the launch of Project Lightspeed, after consulting with his crisis team, Sierk ordered all nonessential BioNTech staff to stay at home.

Uğur, whose concern about infection was reaching new heights, was a step ahead. Weeks earlier, he had abandoned his habit of shaking hands with people at the start of meetings. He was reluctant to even touch papers that needed signing without washing his hands afterward. He emailed BioNTech's operations department asking if an open tent could be procured and built in the parking lot, to enable safer meetings, only to be told this would take a while and was impractical. Long before the rest of the company, he and Özlem, fearing that they would be incapacitated by the virus while the team was most in need of direction, began working from home.

Consisting of just two bedrooms, an all-purpose living/dining room, and a compact annex, the Şahin-Türeci household had felt small before the coronavirus outbreak. Moving to a bigger place had long been on the cards, but Uğur, an avowed urbanite, did not want to relocate to the suburbs, and finding a larger place near their existing home had proved difficult. Now, with Uğur, Özlem, and their daughter all confined to barracks, the apartment felt positively claustrophobic. The teenager was using videoconferencing to keep up with her schoolwork and friends, while her parents continuously joined Zoom meetings with regulators, corporate partners, and suppliers. An internet connection was all that linked the couple to the development of the world's first COVID-19 vaccine.

Most of BioNTech's employees didn't need much convincing to consign themselves to a similar fate. The Mainz campus was already bursting at its seams, with desk space and meeting rooms in short supply. The open-office plans that had been put in place to accommodate new recruits were almost tailor-made to spread disease. When Sierk sent out his decree, the burning question most employees had was not about logistics but timelines. "They asked: 'When will this be over?'" says Sierk, who just replied, "We don't know."

There were still more than five hundred employees, however, who had to be on-site to keep Project Lightspeed going. BioNTech would have to limit the risk of infection as much as possible, but had no experience in drawing up the necessary guidelines. Lab manager François spoke to friends working at Airbus, Bayer, and Nivea maker Beiersdorf. He asked how they were implementing social distancing and similar measures, and he incorporated some of their rules. "We had nothing at the beginning," he says, but the company quickly came up with a scheme to divide essential employees into two groups who would work in separate shifts.

Other than the core scientists, most of those who remained on-site were involved in running or cleaning BioNTech's labs or looking after the manufacturing facilities. The only administrative staffer in the building was Corinna. She had set up a war room in one of the few empty meeting rooms and, with a toddler running around at home, decided to work on campus, even on weekends. Realizing she would be stuck in the office, alone, for most of her waking hours, she brought along a memento from home and placed it on her desk. It was a small painting of a house, by her two-year-old son.

Meanwhile, Alex was working on his pseudovirus test. On March 10, five days after receiving the DNA template at the bus stop, he had a working prototype, but it was far from perfect. The process for detecting whether vaccine-induced antibodies were neutralizing the coronavirus was complex. Healthy cells derived from African green monkeys, which featured the same receptor that the SARS-CoV-2 virus attached to on lung cells, would be placed in small wells resembling those on a muffin tray. Separately, the blood from mice immunized with the vaccine constructs (and hopefully containing neutralizing antibodies) would be mixed with the VSV pseudovirus carrying the coronavirus spike protein and a fluorescent green, glowing enzyme. After an hour or so, the two substances would be combined. If the pseudovirus successfully infected cells—in other words, if antibodies from BioNTech's vaccine *failed* to stop infection—the afflicted cells would glow green under a specialized microscope. If the antibodies in the mouse blood had *successfully* disarmed the coronavirus's spike protein, none, or very few, of the monkey cells would be infected. There would be no green glow.

But the number of cells that would be infected in the absence of antibodies was a tiny fraction of the total in the wells: just five hundred out of forty thousand. When peering down a microscope, it was almost impossible to tell the difference between five hundred infected cells and fifty—to work out how successful the vaccines were. Over the next few weeks Alex and his only colleague, Bianca Sänger, tried to enlist the help of the machines available to them. A flow cytometry device was too slow and the data too noisy. A microplate reader was similarly inaccurate.

In the midst of all this, the Pfizer team, who had just come on board, emailed Annette asking for an SOP—jargon for *standard operating procedure*—of Alex's experiments so that they could attempt to replicate the test in New York. What they wanted was a multipage, step-by-step guide to the process, including details of all the materials, instruments, and techniques involved. When Annette forwarded the request to Alex, he replied with a laughing emoji. There was no such document. Notebooks were not generally taken into labs, to avoid contamination, so like many in his trade, Alex had scribbled his findings on disposable hand towels. Eventually, he would turn them into coherent instructions, but for now—even as Angela Merkel warned Germans they were facing their greatest challenge since World War II[9]—all Alex had to offer one of the world's largest companies was a desk piled high with crumpled tissues.

His method, however, paid off. On March 27, Alex hit the jackpot. A cell-analysis machine the size of a microwave oven, with a highly sensitive fluorescence detector, had delivered the goods. In a matter of minutes, it provided a precise readout of the amount of fluorescent green in all ninety-six wells in his muffin tray. On a laptop, Alex converted this data into a graph, which showed a perfect sigmoidal curve, an elongated S shape, going upward. Here, two months after Uğur had first read about the spread of a strange new pathogen some 8,500 kilometers away, was proof of an mRNA vaccine stripping the coronavirus of its most potent weapon. The antibodies induced by BioNTech's candidates stopped the sometimes-fatal infection in its tracks.

The results were emailed to Uğur, who congratulated the team on their accomplishment. Alex and Bianca celebrated with a high five and immediately got back to work.

Dozens of other samples needed to be tested, and the process remained a precarious one. Larger pharmaceutical companies have several of the cell-analysis devices Alex was using, often sitting idle. BioNTech had one. It was already in high demand for cancer projects, and the device was supposed to be left to cool down for at least ten minutes between each run. Alex contacted the manufacturer, Sartorius, and asked whether doing back-to-back batches would kill the thing. They told him to go ahead and pray it didn't pack up. If it did overheat, they said to give them a call.

Alex and Bianca began working in alternating ten-hour shifts to make the most of the limited amount of time they had with the equipment. Every day, they got closer to burnout, of both human and machine. Eventually, two technicians were seconded to their lab. The team, which had just a few weeks to test whether decades of innovation would pay off, had grown to a sum total of four.

But against all odds, BioNTech was one crucial step closer to creating a viable vaccine. Even Annette, who says she had no doubts that mRNA would meet the moment, admits to having goose bumps when she saw the first readout from the tests of her mice studies. "There was just a small bump in the curve, but it indicated there was something going on," she says. A wave not too dissimilar to those found on a heart monitor indicated, in a new visualization, that antibodies had been brought to the fight. There was no data, as yet, on whether the Lightspeed team's constructs had managed to provoke a T-cell response; the tests were more complicated and would take a while longer to produce results. The company would have to choose a candidate for clinical trials based on Annette and Alex's findings and Uğur and Özlem's well-honed instincts. But in his own way, Uğur marked the occasion. The graph with the little wave became his screen saver.

6

FORGING ALLIANCES

The first Roshni Bhakta heard of a COVID-19 vaccine deal with Pfizer was when a Reuters news flash, in shouty block-capital letters, popped up on her computer screen. An American molecular biologist who had accompanied her German husband back to his homeland, she had been hired by BioNTech after becoming, in her own words, "a mechanic turned car saleswoman" by amassing expertise in patents and licensing. As a scientist, she understood the company's technologies well, and as a canny commercial operator, she knew how to best protect its intellectual property. Her role was becoming increasingly central to BioNTech's business development, as partnerships with drug developers were being inked left and right. Uğur was, by his nature, inclined to trust new collaborators, especially if he saw eye to eye with the researchers involved. Roshni was there to make sure that this trust was not exploited. "My job," she says, "is to protect the company." Which is why the alert on her desktop, on the morning of Friday, March 13, came as a shock.

PFIZER INC—WORKING TO ADVANCE OWN POTENTIAL ANTIVIRAL THERAPIES AND IS ENGAGED WITH BIONTECH ON A POTENTIAL MRNA CORONAVIRUS VACCINE, the news flash read. Roshni, who had just brewed herself a cup of tea, turned around in shock to the only other person in the office that morning, BioNTech's comms chief, Jasmina Alatovic. "Did we . . . ?" she asked. "Did we just do a deal with Pfizer?!" There were only three people in Roshni's department, and none of them had mentioned any upcoming collaboration, save for the one that was in the works with

China's Fosun. Jasmina had not got wind of anything either. This could not be part of the Pfizer flu deal, Roshni knew, as there was no option for the U.S. group to develop further drugs under that agreement.

She did not have to wait long for an answer. By 9:00 a.m., half an hour after the Reuters story was published, an email from Roshni's boss, BioNTech's chief commercial officer, Sean Marett, landed in her inbox. It contained a link to the news agency's article and a one-line instruction: "Please, put a term sheet together." This was corporate-speak for an internal wish list outlining what a collaboration with Pfizer would look like—what rights BioNTech should insist on and what it should offer its partner, financially and scientifically. Roshni immediately began working on the document, and fifteen hours later, at 1:30 a.m. on Saturday, she sent it to Sean.

Once she'd caught her breath, Roshni began to see the logic behind the proposed partnership. While the nature of the announcement had been unorthodox, the move was not wholly unexpected. Ever since Uğur had unveiled his detailed plan for a coronavirus vaccine, it had become increasingly clear to BioNTech's management and senior staff that beyond the initial research and early trials, the company could not go it alone. For a short while, it seemed that international organizations such as the Coalition for Epidemic Preparedness Innovations (CEPI) or the Gates Foundation might step in to help small biotech firms with the latter stages of drug development, securing raw materials, and scaling up manufacturing, but such plans soon disintegrated when confronted with the reality: most companies wanted to do their own thing or partner with their home states. BioNTech would either have to run into the arms of a government, which would then be able to make certain demands, or convince a pharmaceutical giant to give it a helping hand.

Helmut Jeggle, BioNTech's chairman, was in favor of the latter. For an mRNA product to be accepted by the broader population, he felt, one of the beasts of Big Pharma would need to throw its weight behind it. The vaccine would also have to be transported worldwide in ultra-freezing temperatures, at least for the initial rollout, and BioNTech would need the assistance of a corporation used to handling complex logistics. Partnering with a larger company would also provide a level of protection against litigation, especially in the U.S., where "no win, no fee" lawyers would inevitably coax a handful of disgruntled patients into launching a legal challenge against any new drugmaker, especially one relying on a novel technology.

More importantly, however, Helmut knew BioNTech needed to accelerate. He believed that for the investment into Project Lightspeed to pay off, its vaccine had to be among the first three to come to market, while global demand was still high. To do this, the German company would need to demonstrate to regulators in a matter of months that its candidate had an outstanding efficacy and safety profile in enormous Phase 3 trials, involving tens of thousands of people across several countries. Only five manufacturers were capable of carrying out a global vaccine study of that scale and speed: Merck, Johnson & Johnson, Sanofi, GlaxoSmithKline, and Pfizer. One of them was already working with BioNTech.

The path forward seemed obvious. But for Uğur and Özlem, it was not an easy one to take. Bitter experience had taught them that such a route could be riddled with trade-offs.

The couple's independence, and consequently BioNTech's, was hard won. The company's very existence was down to their determination to prioritize scientific excellence over short-term profits. They had been saved from falling prey to pharmaceutical giants by a pair of Bavarian billionaires in search of a breakthrough to back and bequeath to their families. It was a privileged position that Uğur and Özlem had always been loath to risk at the hands of an opportunistic partner.

The doctors' early experience of the commercial world had been a chastening one. After being repeatedly rebuffed by large drug developers, Uğur and Özlem had decided to spin off their own company from their university research groups in Mainz and Zurich "out of desperation," says Özlem. Watching American biotechs with a single conceptual product enjoy enormous financial support, the duo decided they had to go it alone if they were ever to see their many innovations administered to patients.

But the year was 2001, and their timing could not have been worse.

Germany was reeling from the bursting of the dot-com bubble, exemplified by the collapse of the country's Neuer Markt index, which had been created as a rival to New York's tech-focused Nasdaq. Risk-averse investors in the country, who had been coaxed into backing a handful of tech darlings, lost fortunes and vowed never to be caught up in such hype again. Even in more bullish times, mainland Europe was not a particularly hospitable environment for biotech companies. There were only a handful of investment funds paying attention to the sector and even fewer analysts offering regular coverage of relevant start-ups. "At some point, we understood there was no other way," Özlem says, so the couple began searching for backers interested in a business that would focus on monoclonal antibodies, a relatively well-established form of cancer treatment. Uğur, who had never wanted to start his own firm, likened their mission to that of hobbit Frodo Baggins in one of his favorite fantasy movies, *The Lord of the Rings*. Frodo did not choose to be the ring bearer, he told Özlem, nor to be responsible for its destruction, but was forced to take on the task.

It would not be an easy sell. Uğur's and Özlem's profiles were not particularly attractive to domestic investors. Germany had virtually no prominent entrepreneurs from an immigrant background, and Uğur and Özlem lacked the sheen that came with a stint at a prestigious U.S. university, such as Harvard or Johns Hopkins. This was a route typically taken by the most ambitious scientists in the country, and venture capitalists held the *in Amerika gewesen* (those who have been in America) in far higher regard than those who chose to stay put. But the strength of the couple's research, and Özlem's ability to explain it in eloquent German, won over some skeptics. Eventually, they managed to raise 7 million deutschemarks (around €3.6 million) from a Swiss investor, becoming the only start-up in the country to do so that year. They called their company Ganymed, a name plucked from a line in a poem by Goethe, which sounds similar to the Turkish expression for *hard-earned*.

In the early years of Ganymed, Uğur and Özlem found the journey to be far less perilous than that of their hobbit role model's. Then, in 2007, the couple and their mentor, the Austrian oncologist Christoph Huber, who had cofounded Ganymed with them six years earlier, suddenly found themselves with their backs against the wall. The start-up had several preclinical accomplishments under its belt and was preparing for its first human trials after two financing rounds. But Ganymed now needed to invest in costly, large-scale studies, and it had run out of money. Nextech, a Zurich-based venture capital firm that had provided the seed capital for the company and remained its largest investor, wanted out. Uğur and Özlem understood that the firm had internal rules on how long individual companies could remain under its wing, and Nextech now needed to exit, to recoup what it could from its investment.

Uğur and Özlem, who in the intervening years had gained some business expertise, knew this meant that one of three things would happen: they would be forced to merge with another biotech; Ganymed would be flogged in a fire sale; or, in the worst-case scenario, they would be forced to file for insolvency, leaving their precious patents in the hands of liquidators. Finding new funders also seemed out of the question—who would pick up a company that had been all but discarded by its previous owners? But as luck would have it, the trio had recently been introduced to a pair of extremely enthusiastic, and unorthodox, investors. Having made their money by selling a generic drugs giant, Hexal, in a $7.5 billion deal, these entrepreneurs had put a small amount—a couple of million euros—into Ganymed and seemed disappointed not to be able to buy a bigger stake. If anyone could get them out of this predicament, Uğur and Özlem realized, it was the Strüngmann twins: Thomas and Andreas.

In September 2007, running out of options, the couple and Christoph Huber traveled to Munich, where, in a conference room at the Strüngmanns' office overlooking a busy, tram-lined road, they described their dilemma. Seated opposite them was Thomas Strüngmann, the more affable of the almost identical brothers, and his advisor Helmut Jeggle, who was in charge of the family's investments. Michael Motschmann, the head of a smaller investment fund called MIG, was alongside them. He had brought Uğur and Özlem's biotech company to the attention of Thomas a few months earlier during a round of golf played on the picturesque shores of Bavaria's Lake Tegernsee.

During the discussion in Munich, Helmut revealed that while the

Strüngmanns' office had considered upping its stake in Ganymed, the company's Swiss backers, along with institutional investors such as Germany's state-owned development bank, KfW, had indicated that they would not allow their majority share to be diluted, effectively tying Thomas's hands. But doing nothing, he knew, threatened to bring Uğur and Özlem's entrepreneurial streak to a halt. Companies, Thomas was fond of saying, were only as good as their people, and he was reluctant to let these particular people leave his orbit. "I was fascinated by them," he says. "I thought, 'This is the couple that will fulfill our dreams.'" He turned to Uğur and Özlem and asked, "If Ganymed were to implode, do you have anything else up your sleeve?"

Uğur paused. He and Özlem had been quietly working on several projects, including mRNA therapies, with their small group of scientists at the Mainz university and were already entertaining the idea of launching a second business—one devoted to a handful of next-generation platforms that could help cancer patients through individualized drugs targeted at tumors. But having been rattled by Nextech's planned departure, and having seen their stakes in Ganymed already reduced to less than 1.5 percent each, Uğur and Özlem were reluctant to be beholden to outsiders once again. As one pharma exec had warned them, biotechs were built to die; they disappeared either by acquisition or, far more often, by failure. The couple's other projects, code-named NT, for New Technologies, were too dear to their hearts to be allowed to suffer such a fate. They could, Uğur believed, be funded with the sale of Ganymed, along with grants from the German government. It would not be the sort of money that enabled the new company to get a product to market within a few years, but NT would be able to trundle along, slowly but surely, without the background noise of regular financing rounds and pitches to fund managers.

Reluctantly, however, they began presenting some of their recent work to the investors in the Strüngmanns' office, including mRNA cancer therapies as well as a library of tumor-specific antigens that the couple had discovered using an early version of artificial intelligence and which could be used to target cancer cells. These were early innovations, they stressed, and investing in them would carry a great risk. "We made it clear that it would take ten years for these technologies to be realized," says Uğur. The couple wanted to build an immunotherapy company like no other, he told the meeting, investigating everything from mRNA to cell and gene therapies, to biospecific antibodies and immunomodulators. They couldn't, and wouldn't, commit to timelines for clinical trials. Instead, they would test their innovations in humans once *they* judged them ready, rather than to fit the financing cycles of investors.

Despite these stipulations, Thomas was getting excited. An economist by training, he had developed some scientific expertise by learning from his father, who had founded his own pharmaceutical business, and his twin brother, Andreas, a medical doctor. He was vaguely aware of the skepticism surrounding mRNA platforms, but it was in his nature to back a shunned horse, particularly if the investment required was modest, relative to the family's recently acquired wealth. He had made enough money to make some mistakes and could afford to rely, at least in part, on his instincts. "I didn't understand very much of it at that time," he readily admits, "but I had a gut feeling."

Once Uğur and Özlem had concluded their presentation, Thomas, who was not yet on first-name terms with the couple, turned to them. "Professor Şahin; Dr. Türeci, how much money do you need for this?" he asked matter-of-factly. Unprepared, the doctors quickly calculated what it would cost to get to the point where they could launch a couple of Phase 2 clinical trials within half a decade. To do so, they told the group, they would need roughly €150 million. Thomas jumped to his feet and asked to be excused from the room to make a phone call.

A few minutes later, having called Andreas, Thomas returned. "Well, you have the money," he announced. A bemused Uğur and Özlem looked at each other, and then at Christoph and Michael, who were equally taken aback. Supporting an entirely new venture, they knew, would be highly unusual for the Strüngmanns' investment vehicle, known by its trade name, Athos. The fund was not in the habit of providing seed capital—it preferred to invest once a young company already had its corporate scaffolding in place. Plus, the brothers had been concerned that if Özlem and Uğur left Ganymed—in which they had already invested—to focus on a new firm, the company would lose all direction and fetch even less in a fire sale. But Thomas, enthused by the duo's impromptu presentation, was convinced that they were just a few years away from upending the pharma world. To underline his commitment, he said, Athos would guarantee that the doctors could concentrate on their new venture, uninterrupted, for five years, without having to worry about bank balances. At the end of that period, Thomas and Helmut believed that Uğur and Özlem's company would have created enough value to raise significantly more money. Until then, along with a small contribution from MIG, the Strüngmanns would put down the €150 million. They were all in.

Özlem, Uğur, and Christoph, however, were not celebrating just yet. They were adamant that the company soon to be known as BioNTech, incorporating the project name NT, would only be built on their terms. The tables had turned; now it was Athos that would have to do the pitching to three jaded entrepreneurs. "I told them we were a family office; we weren't constantly looking at the return on investment," Helmut Jeggle remembers. Detecting that the couple were still skeptical, Thomas Strüngmann made an unrefusable offer. He would agree to a no-questions-asked clause, meaning the brothers would not interfere in the company's affairs for at least a couple of years, and the trio would be free to go in whichever direction they liked. Upon Uğur's request, and to show that they were in it for the long run, Athos also agreed to forfeit the right to force a sale until 2023—giving BioNTech fifteen years of stability, breathing room that would be beyond the wildest dreams of most founders.

In the ensuing weeks, however, the creation of the new company was complicated by the fact that Nextech had, after all, agreed to part with its stake in Ganymed. Now the Strüngmanns were of two minds—should they invest in Ganymed and simultaneously fund BioNTech? Could the couple manage both? Thomas was in favor of the more adventurous option: buying out the existing Ganymed investors, putting in Özlem as chief executive, and pumping enough money into the company to make it an attractive asset for a potential buyer. "If you tell Thomas it will get much warmer if you go a little bit south, he will go south," says Helmut

Jeggle. But Andreas was less convinced, and by April, Uğur was having second thoughts too.

To clear the air, the brothers arranged a meeting at a private retreat in the Taunus, a bucolic mountain range just north of Frankfurt that is home to many of the city's wealthiest. The Villa Rothschild was built in 1888 as summer residence for Wilhelm Carl von Rothschild, the scion of Frankfurt's famous banking dynasty, who used it to entertain nobility from around the world. Over the next 120 years, the property became a magnet for great thinkers and leaders, especially during the late 1940s, when parts of Germany's constitution had been drafted on-site. The historic significance of the location was not lost on Uğur and Özlem as they sat in the foyer of the neo-baronial building with Thomas, Michael, and Helmut. Drinking tea and surveying the area's lush rolling hills through the hotel's enormous bay windows, it was easy to see why so many important people had been attracted to this elevated spot. Perhaps, they thought as they went through their draft agreement for BioNTech line by line, deals of far more significance had been hashed out in this very room and sealed with a clink of a sherry glass.

Such a scenario was not on the cards for the two scientists just yet. While they had reached a compromise with the Strüngmanns on almost every outstanding issue, the couple's benefactors balked at Uğur's suggested valuation for BioNTech of €70 million, along with the demand that he and Özlem retain 25 percent of the business. Unable to reach an accord, Helmut suggested a walk.

As they strolled through the villa's verdant grounds, Uğur and Helmut made a concerted effort not to talk shop. Instead, they made awkward conversation about their surroundings and their families, all the while realizing that if they returned to the hotel without an agreement, it would likely be curtains for this partnership. Time, they both knew, was of the essence. Without waiting for the Strüngmanns' cash, Uğur had already hired a few scientists for the as-yet-unnamed BioNTech and was financing their salaries out of his own pocket. He was fast running out of money and confessed to Helmut that he was just four weeks from being unable to pay his skeleton staff.

By the time they reached the small lake that formed the centerpiece of the estate's gardens, Helmut was ready to make a proposal. Standing on a bridge, he turned to Uğur. "Come on, let's do a deal. We'll give you 20 percent, and we will put 5 percent aside. If everything goes well after five years, Thomas will give you that 5 percent." He stretched out his hand. Uğur clasped it, but came up with an alternative suggestion: "Let's do it the other way around: I'll take 25 percent, and if we fail, I'll give the 5 percent back." Helmut, unable to disguise his admiration for Uğur's newfound business savvy, smiled and promised to do what he could to convince his employers.

When they walked back into the hotel, the pair paused underneath an oil painting depicting some of the architects of Germany's Basic Law, who had gathered at the Villa Rothschild in the aftermath of World War II, hoping to set the country on a path to renewal. Neither Uğur nor Helmut, who were still in the process of getting properly acquainted, dared speak their thoughts out loud. Carried away with emotion, they imagined that one day another artwork might hang alongside it, portraying the moment BioNTech was born.

On June 2, 2008, BioNTech was founded in Mainz to zero fanfare. A few weeks later, Lehman Brothers collapsed, and the world was plunged into a financial crisis.

Thanks to the Strüngmanns' up-front investment, BioNTech was able to carry on regardless. A couple of months after signing the deal with the Bavarian brothers, the company agreed to buy a peptide manufacturer in Berlin for €3 million to give it easy access to crucial raw materials and decrease its dependence on other manufacturers. After one year, thanks to a string of further acquisitions, Uğur and Özlem's fledgling business had grown to three hundred staff.

All the while, BioNTech had purposely remained virtually anonymous. "We built the company according to our vision, brick by brick,"

Uğur explains. "For others, what we wanted to do sounded like science fiction. Experienced pharmaceutical experts ridiculed us for the idea of wanting to develop individualized immunotherapies, and we had no reason to advertise our concepts." BioNTech would have no presence at biotech conferences over the next five years. Its website would feature a lone banner, reading: "Under Construction."

The focus was on getting on with cutting-edge research and development with minimal disruption. Uğur and Özlem continued to pursue a broad range of cutting-edge technologies and built up their manufacturing expertise. But there were setbacks along the way. In 2011, Uğur had told the company's supervisory board that they faced a choice. The team that had grown out of his and Özlem's lab had significantly improved the potency of mRNA, and they had a cancer treatment that was ready to go into clinic, which they believed would ultimately gain regulatory approval. But Uğur felt that with a few more years' work, the immune responses triggered by the molecule could be increased by a factor of one hundred. All he wanted was some more time.

Once again, the Strüngmanns gave their blessing and on several subsequent occasions opted to wait for a technological breakthrough rather than monetize the perfectly passable prototypes BioNTech had already developed. Thomas remembers the period as a steep learning curve. If you invest in early-stage biotechs, he discovered, "it always costs much more than you planned for and takes longer than you thought." In the end, the Strüngmanns, who also founded a neuroscience institute in memory of their father, would double their investment into BioNTech to fund iterative cycles of improvement. Without this cash, the company would not have had the time to develop mature mRNA platforms, which several years later allowed it to create twenty COVID-19 vaccine candidates within a matter of weeks.

Five years after BioNTech's founding, however, in 2013, the Phase 2 studies Uğur and Özlem had promised the Strüngmanns were still nowhere to be seen. Other pharmaceutical executives were beginning to urge Helmut to pull Athos's funds; the company, one warned, would "only burn money." BioNTech's biggest competitors were beginning to outpace the scientists in Mainz, or at least that is what it seemed like to outsiders. In March 2013, the Anglo-Swedish drug giant AstraZeneca announced an agreement with mRNA firm Moderna, which included an up-front payment of $240 million. Months later, the biotech received a further $25 million from DARPA, an offshoot of the U.S. Department of Defense. Closer to home, Germany's CureVac had signed deals with Johnson & Johnson, France's Sanofi, and the Gates Foundation.

BioNTech's investors were eager to do similar deals. There was simply not enough cash to fund each of Uğur and Özlem's ideas all the way to the clinic. External funds would soon be needed, and they wanted an indication of what their company's innovations were now worth to the market. Reluctantly, Uğur agreed to allow Sean Marett, whose skills as a salesman had been honed on the UK biotech scene as well as at Big Pharma's GlaxoSmithKline, to begin spying out the land.

The biopharmaceutical industry, it turned out, was slowly beginning to recognize the value of BioNTech's proprietary technologies. After attending every medical conference that would let him in, from Japan to Europe to the U.S., Sean finally sealed the company's first agreement in 2015, with Indianapolis-based Eli Lilly. The American company agreed to put in a total of $60 million,[1] in return for the ability to license potential cancer immunotherapy drugs. Larger and increasingly lucrative deals followed, with Denmark's Genmab, then Sanofi. This time, however, at Uğur's urging, they were fifty-fifty partnerships. BioNTech would not readily give up its independence, he insisted, and a trickle of takeover attempts via bankers were instantly rebuffed by the board.

This approach raised eyebrows among industry veterans. In 2015, when Sean related BioNTech's plans to Merck's then CEO Roger Perlmutter, the executive, who had been at a smaller start-up himself, was taken aback. He warned Sean that self-reliance would be harder work than he imagined. Within weeks, however, BioNTech had begun negotiations with the most successful of all biotechs, San Francisco's Genentech, treated almost as a deity in Silicon Valley circles. By September 2016, the company, which had been acquired by Switzerland's Roche, agreed to pay $310 million up front to secure an equal partnership with BioNTech. Despite his disdain for Big

Pharma, Uğur saw this as an opportunity. He already knew Ira Mellman, a highly respected immunologist who worked at Genentech, and the two shared many of the same scientific beliefs. Due to this relationship, Uğur was open to exploring whether BioNTech could leverage Roche's global clinical network to get lifesaving treatments to market quickly and learn from observing that process. Crucially, the company would also benefit from having to develop its own commercial expertise, which it could use to limit the number of collaborations it entered into in the future.

Meanwhile, Özlem, who had cofounded BioNTech with Uğur and Christoph Huber and helped in an informal capacity at every step, still held no official role at that company. Her unique talents were needed elsewhere, specifically at the trio's first firm, Ganymed, which had reached a critical stage in the typical biotech's life cycle. It would soon seek to prove its core concepts in a randomized human trial, comparing how its product performed against existing cancer treatments. Half of the original management team had moved on, with Uğur going to BioNTech, and as a result, it had been reduced to a two-person operation: Özlem—the only person with the necessary scientific *and* business expertise to get Ganymed over this line—was serving as chief executive and chief medical officer, supported by Dirk Sebastian, who had been at the start-up since its inception and took responsibility for the finances. Despite having too few hands on deck, Ganymed's first Phase 2 study delivered more impressive results than Uğur and Özlem had ever dared to dream of. "It was a game changer because it validated us as clinical innovators," says Özlem. In participants with a certain type of gastric cancer, the combination of standard chemotherapy and Ganymed's new antibody treatment managed to both shrink tumors and prevent them from regrowing. The patients' chances of survival nearly doubled.

This encouraging data catapulted Ganymed into the international limelight. The company was showcased prominently at ASCO, the world's biggest cancer conference, and major news outlets, including *Fortune* magazine, asked why no one had heard of this "obscure biotech" with a potential "game-changing cancer med." Several companies suddenly wanted to buy Ganymed, and an offer from Japan's Astellas proved too good to pass up. In 2016, the Strüngmanns agreed to sell the business for $1.4 billion in Germany's biggest biotech deal. In one fell swoop, the brothers' investments in Uğur and Özlem's start-ups had paid off. Handsomely.

The transaction proved bittersweet for Özlem. She had hoped to get the treatment to market via an accelerated approval path so that patients around the world might benefit from it while a Phase 3 trial was being conducted, rather than having to wait for its conclusion. Instead, she and her team went through an extensive handover process with Astellas, which ultimately decided to embark on its own large-scale global trials that, as of the end of 2021, remain ongoing.

Now that Ganymed had been sold, however, Özlem was free to join BioNTech's board. With several deals on the horizon, the core investors wanted her to take on the role of chief medical officer, to shepherd the company's many disparate technologies into the clinic. Reluctant to repeat her experience at Ganymed and "lose another baby," Özlem hesitated. "After we sold Ganymed, I was very disappointed," she says. "It seemed that conventional biotech business models and financing mechanisms were an obstacle to moving innovations to patients' bedsides."

Uğur, Helmut, Christoph Huber, and Thomas Strüngmann, among many others, did their best to persuade her otherwise. "This time, it will be different," Uğur told her. "BioNTech will reinvent the model." For their part, the Strüngmanns underlined their commitment to developing a stand-alone company, rather than one that would be sold to a larger rival. Their firm determination, along with Uğur's, convinced Özlem that, as in the past, they would figure it out together, on the go. She agreed to come on board, but knowing there were tough years ahead, she bought herself a gold pendant as a welcome gift. Inscribed on one side of the necklace, which she wears to this day, were the words *Grow Grit,* and on the other, *Spartan Up!*

Although partnerships and collaborations were now being signed frequently by BioNTech, further funding proved hard to come by. Foreign biotech companies were almost invisible in the U.S.—where most potential investors were based. "We lacked the name recognition," says chief strategy officer Ryan Richardson, who at the time was looking at the bio-tech industry with an investment banker's glasses. Plus, money managers would normally only invest in one experimental mRNA start-up, and many had already funded Moderna, whose smooth-talking French chief executive, Stéphane Bancel, had done a good job of wooing Wall Street. In 2016, before Sean flew to New York for a health care conference run by Citigroup, he submitted dozens of meeting requests on the event's online "speed dating" system, designed to connect interesting companies with interested investors. Only a lone "strategy and corporate communications advisor" would have coffee with him.

Frustrated, Sean, whose Cockney twang gives him a Ray Winstone–esque charisma, called the offices of Manhattan-based fund managers and begged for half an hour of their time while he was in town. On a snowy December week, the stubble-bearded executive trudged from building to building on Madison Avenue, armed with a presentation that explained how BioNTech had risen to be Germany's largest unlisted bio-tech, with hundreds of employees and a plethora of partnerships under its belt. Founders Uğur and Özlem, he explained, had recently published three times in *Nature,* one of a handful of elite scientific journals. In response, he was met with blank stares, and sometimes a ruder version of: "Who the hell are you, and why are you wasting my time?"

The reception in Europe was even frostier. In April 2017, Sean attended a conference in Amsterdam, where in a small room on the banks of one of the city's canals, the sharp-talking Englishman suggested that BioNTech—which would be more valuable than Deutsche Bank by the end of 2020—was already worth €2 billion, making it one of Europe's precious few billion-euro start-ups, or unicorns. The room erupted with laughter. During the coffee break following his presentation, a friend sidled up to him. "They're talking about you," he said, pointing to a group of suited male managers huddled in a corner, "and they think you are crazy." Unperturbed, Sean, who was looking to raise €300 million, would not budge on what he believed to be a fair sticker price, particularly given the eye-watering valuations for American companies with much less to show for their efforts. "That's when I realized, we were never going to get any money in Europe—ever—from professional funds," he says, "and so I spent my time in the U.S."

Uğur, who loathed pitching, largely left Sean to do the fundraising. When investors asked to speak to BioNTech's founders, he would struggle to explain his boss's absence, and although he had studied biochemistry, Sean occasionally found himself stuck on the science. At a meeting in Denver that May, fund managers started peppering him with questions on one of Uğur and Özlem's publications. He tried valiantly to answer them, but stumbled, to the irritation of his inquisitors. "See, if you want to get an American investor, you really have to know all the answers," a gruff manager warned him.

An unlikely breakthrough came a few months later, in September 2017, when a big black coach with tinted windows pulled up outside the company's Mainz headquarters. Its passengers were fund managers assembled by Credit Suisse for a bus tour around Europe to scope out biotech investment opportunities, and BioNTech was added as a stop at the last minute, after Sean had surreptitiously talked to the organizers.

The night before the fund managers' arrival, Sean had been entertaining executives from BioNTech's partner Genentech at Munich's Oktoberfest beer festival and was now battling a severe hangover. To make matters worse, Uğur was supposed to present a series of slides, but, still not a fan of meeting investors, spontaneously decided to dispense with formalities and proceeded directly to a question-and-answer session. What followed was akin to a prolonged quick-fire round on a TV quiz show. For two hours, seasoned pharma investors bombarded Uğur with queries. Patiently, he walked them through the decades of research that underpinned BioNTech's advances, in the same über-rationalist manner in which he and Özlem had convinced the Strüngmanns to part with their cash years earlier. After he had finished, a representative of institutional investor Fidelity made a beeline for Sean. He had heard the company was considering launching its first funding round, he said. "Is there any room for us?"

On the back of that afternoon's performance, BioNTech raised $270[2] million, in the sixth-largest series A, or initial financing round, for a biotech worldwide. The money allowed the company to build the production fa-cilities in Mainz that would end up manufacturing crucial COVID-19 vaccine doses for clinical trials in early 2020. An even larger round fol-lowed in July 2019, when BioNTech managed to bring in a further $325 million, mostly from existing backers. The figure accounted for 61 per-cent of all investment in German biotechs in 2019.[3] Soon, it was time for the ultimate step, going public on a stock exchange, and opening the company up to investors the world over.

BioNTech's timing, however, was less than fortuitous. In the sum-mer of 2019, as board members flew in a chartered plane from one American city to another to drum up interest for their IPO, the Nas-daq's biotechnology index, on which the company planned to list, hit rock bottom. Investors were spooked by the U.S.-China trade war, overvalued stocks, and the prospect of a looming recession. Both the ride-hailing app Uber and fitness-equipment maker Peloton had strug-gled in their recent public debuts, and a week before BioNTech was supposed to go public, another European health start-up, ADC Ther-apeutics,[4] pulled its flotation, citing unfavorable market conditions. On a mobile app provided by BioNTech's lead bankers, J. P. Morgan, the traveling circus of Uğur, Sean, Helmut, and business development manager Holger Kissel could check in regularly to see precisely how few of the investors they met on their whirlwind tour had subscribed to reserve shares in the company, in the so-called book-building process that precedes an IPO. Disheartened, they considered postponement. Sean, however, was eager to plow ahead, and in the end BioNTech raised just $150 million, at a valuation of $3.5 billion, roughly $100 million less than it had hoped to fetch.

Still, the IPO served its main purpose: announcing BioNTech to the world. After ringing the bell in New York to open the day's trad-ing on the morning of the company's listing, under the ticker symbol BNTX, Uğur and Özlem walked out into Times Square with their teen-age daughter to see their other baby's name in lights. BioNTech's logo was plastered all over the digital billboards that lined the Nasdaq sky-scraper, with the tagline: "Every patient's cancer is unique." The mes-sage they had delivered to the Strüngmanns all those years ago was finally getting through. New Technologies had gone from a pet project to the eighth German company ever to list on the same exchange as Microsoft, Apple, and Google.

Being under the full glare of the open market, however, had its drawbacks. BioNTech would now have to update investors on its progress every three months, define targets, and explain if and why it had missed them. Plus, the lackluster listing in New York had left the company needing to raise more money to fund the development of its drugs. In its filing for the IPO, BioNTech had provided a hint to its future: "We currently have no marketing and sales organization, and as a company, we have no experience in marketing pharmaceutical products. If we are unable to establish marketing and sales capabilities on our own or through third parties, we may not be able to market and sell our product candidates effectively in the United States and other jurisdictions, if approved, or generate product sales revenue."[5] Unlike Moderna, BioNTech had not drawn on large grants from the U.S. government,[6] and going it alone was not an option. Tie-ups with Big Pharma were almost inevitable.

That moment came sooner than expected. In February 2020, seated round the table in Uğur's office, BioNTech's supervisory board realized that to get a COVID-19 vaccine to market in record time, they would have to accept the embrace of a larger firm, even if it risked seeing their greatest accomplishment to date, and their first-ever commercial product, become forever associated with another household brand. Pfizer was the obvious choice.

Just three years earlier, the U.S. pharma giant was at the bottom of BioNTech's list of potential partners. Sean would meet Pfizer executives regularly at the health care conferences he attended and found the company impossible to navigate. Representatives from Pfizer's West Coast team wanted to know about cell and gene therapies, while its New York managers always asked about a completely different technology: antibody sequences. Pfizer did not seem to be a well-coordinated organization.

Nonetheless, Sean persisted and in 2013 tried to convince the corporation to help BioNTech develop a flu jab that would provide more protection than existing vaccines, which in some years were less than 50 percent effective at preventing severe disease. Initial meetings at Pfizer's headquarters on Manhattan's East Forty-second Street took place in small "collaboration pods," which sat just three people and had gray curtains that could be drawn to create the illusion of privacy. Eight such meetings, mostly with middle managers, took place over the next four years, and the project progressed so slowly that Sean soon stopped flying over to attend them, sending Holger instead.

In November 2017, when Pfizer asked to meet with BioNTech at a conference called BIO-Europe, Holger went along to that too. All of a sudden, there was a sense of urgency from the company, which was especially interested in BioNTech's small, but growing, infectious disease pipeline. Sean knew the U.S. drugmaker had already been in discussion with CureVac and that BioNTech was late to the game. But Pfizer seemed keener than ever. Video calls between the companies' science teams followed, and a delegation from Pfizer's U.S. base flew over to Mainz to inspect BioNTech's headquarters. Among the visitors was Phil Dormitzer, Pfizer's chief scientific officer for viral vaccines, who had significant mRNA expertise and who would be Uğur's first port of call in February 2020 to float the idea of working on a COVID-19 vaccine. Phil was impressed by the range of BioNTech's technologies. "Their philosophy was: 'We will look at everything,'" he recalls. "It became clear that scientifically, we were very compatible."

In the autumn, Sean got a call from Holger, who had received an abnormal reception during yet another meeting at Pfizer's skyscraper in New York. The company's head of external innovation had attended and brought along his entire team. The executive was straightforward: he wanted to know if BioNTech was ready to collaborate on a flu product. "I think they are serious this time," Holger told Sean over the phone shortly afterward. "There were eight people in the pod."

The next week, when Sean flew to New York for follow-up meetings, he discovered why Pfizer had suddenly accelerated their approach. A young researcher in the company's business development division had read a series of papers by Uğur and Özlem in *Nature* and forwarded them to her higher-ups. One of those was Kathrin Jansen, a German-born microbiologist who had led the development of the world's first cervical cancer jab and had been rewarded with the top job in Pfizer's vaccine research unit. Like Phil, she appreciated the fact that in contrast to some other mRNA companies she had vetted, BioNTech was "interested in keeping an open mind." Kathrin also liked the fact that the company was not an infectious diseases specialist and did not come with preconceived ideas. At her command, negotiations gathered pace, and in February 2018, a meeting was arranged with Uğur in New York.

Holger, who stayed behind in Mainz, did his best to prepare Uğur for the occasion. Phil also warned Uğur that Kathrin would be very critical and direct. Panic began to set in when Uğur, who had just emerged from a disappointing meeting with France's Sanofi at their U.S. headquarters in New Jersey, called to say he wasn't feeling very well. Nonetheless, he kept his appointment with Kathrin, with Holger dialed in from Germany. Her staff, eager for the encounter to go well, had suggested to Holger that Uğur kick off the meeting with a few sentences in German, to strike up a kinship, which he duly did. The cultural connection did not prevent Uğur's compatriot from giving him a tough time. "She really, in a German way, challenged me," he recalls.

"I played the skeptic," says Kathrin. "I explained to him that I had come through the time of DNA vaccines and it had not been a particularly good experience," she recalls. The technology was touted as "the solution for everything," but turned out to be a false dawn.

For twenty minutes, Kathrin laid out the reasons why mRNA drugs would not work, to which Uğur responded, one by one. "All her questions were fair," he says, "but she made it very clear from the very beginning that she needs to be convinced." Once his inquisitor was satisfied, the tables were turned, and Kathrin began to pitch to Uğur—explaining why Pfizer and BioNTech would make a good match. She made it clear that the American company was serious about actually using mRNA technology, rather than buying into it as a hedge, to sit on a shelf, out of competitors' reach. After another meeting in New York, the two began to develop some chemistry. "We hit it off because we are both science driven," says Kathrin, who agreed to collaborate with Uğur on an mRNA flu vaccine. In a departure from BioNTech's attempts to maintain control of all its products, Pfizer would manufacture and license this jab, paying royalties to its junior partner. An agreement was drawn up, and in July 2018, the deal was signed.

By February 2020, the groundwork for further collaboration had been laid. There were four meetings a year between the companies, two in the U.S. and two in Germany, to review the flu partnership's progress. Uğur, Özlem, and their daughter had been to dinner with Kathrin and her husband when they came over from New York to visit Mainz, and the families developed a friendship. Senior BioNTech staff involved in the influenza program knew their counterparts at Pfizer well.

Even after Phil Dormitzer rebuffed Uğur's first approach, declining to jointly develop a vaccine for the coronavirus, which he believed would largely be confined to China, the BioNTech board continued to pin their hopes on Pfizer, which, due to the established relationship, was best placed to join Project Lightspeed with minimum fuss. As the prospect of a Phase 3 trial, involving tens of thousands of people, loomed, the board was increasingly aware of the fact that it had neither the finances, nor the territorial coverage, to even contemplate going solo. "There was always an element of: this is a global problem and requires a global solution," says Ryan. "We needed a strong U.S. ally, and we needed a strong Chinese ally."

The latter was proving an easier sell, with Shanghai-based Fosun, whose executives were witnessing the epidemic firsthand, showing an ever-keener interest in a collaboration. Slowly, the virus was strengthening the argument for a partnership with Pfizer too. Italy's Lombardy region was seeing hundreds of new cases each day, and its hospitals were struggling to cope. Doctors in the U.S. were already pleading for tougher travel restrictions as cases in the country spread from Washington to Florida. In California's Santa Clara County, dozens of people were dying with COVID-19-like symptoms, although this would not be publicly confirmed for a few more weeks.[7] The number of deaths worldwide was creeping up to three thousand,[8] more than the total number of fatalities from the first SARS virus and MERS combined. Perhaps by now, Uğur reasoned, the American group would share his belief that this disease was not going to vanish overnight.

On March 3, Uğur called Kathrin directly with a renewed pitch. This time, the reception was markedly different. Before he could finish his argument for extending BioNTech and Pfizer's alliance to a COVID-19 vaccine, Kathrin interrupted. "I said, 'Perfect,' because mRNA ticked all the boxes," she remembers. "There was no doubt in my mind [that it was the right technology for this task]." In principle, the 170-year-old company was on board.

A few days later, Albert Bourla, a Greek vet who had worked his way up the Pfizer corporate ladder for a quarter of a century before becoming chief executive in 2019, was in his home country waiting to speak at the Delphi Economic Forum. He received a note saying the conference, due to begin on March 5, had suddenly been canceled. "That was a big alert for me," says Albert.[9] He had already tasked a team at Pfizer with exploring the possibility of developing a COVID-19 therapeutic, after discussions with Mikael Dolsten, Pfizer's chief scientific officer. Unaware of the call between Phil and Uğur in February, he had also asked staff to look at whether the company, one of the world's "big four" vaccine producers, had the capability to create a coronavirus shot.

"The team came back suggesting mRNA," he remembers, "which was a surprise to me, because it was not a proven technology." Albert's involvement in the influenza project with BioNTech had been minimal; he had first seen the deal when it came to his desk for approval in 2018. "I was not paying particular attention," he readily admits, "and I did not know Uğur or anyone else at this time." When a coronavirus collaboration with BioNTech was suggested by Kathrin, Albert asked to speak to Uğur himself, and a call between the two was hastily arranged. "It was love at first sight," the Pfizer chief executive says of their first discussion, "a great meeting of the minds." Very quickly, he says, "I established that Uğur was a very honest, inspiring man—the element of trust was unusually high." For his part, Uğur says he found Albert to be "really informed and personally engaged."

After some small talk, the two chief executives moved on to basic ground rules. "I was concerned that if we went into a partnership with Pfizer, the project could be slowed down because risk-averse companies want to see more data before progressing to the next stage," Uğur says. "It was important to me to define principles, one of which was that if one party wanted to go ahead at any point, the other could not stop it." Another principle was that BioNTech would maintain its independence, for which Uğur and Özlem had fought after the Ganymed experience and had won thanks to the Strüngmanns. Unlike with the flu vaccine, this would be a fifty-fifty deal, Uğur proposed. There would be no David and Goliath in this arrangement. The companies would share the costs and potential profits equally.

Recalling this conversation over a year later, Albert says he had no objections to this setup. He does not know if others in Pfizer were pushing for a more traditional licensing agreement, "but for me, fifty-fifty was always fine." If the companies were successful, there would be more than enough of a yield to go around. If they failed, they would have bigger problems than their respective bank balances. The world would be in serious trouble.

With the fundamentals out of the way, Uğur and Albert began to discuss timelines. Normally, such an agreement entails line-by-line contract negotiations between business development teams and corporate and patent lawyers and takes at least half a year to complete. Faced with a looming pandemic, both bosses agreed that BioNTech and Pfizer did not have such luxuries. "We had a discussion in which we said we need to start immediately," says Albert, "and then let the paperwork come whenever it comes." He had already told his staff not to spend a second worrying about budgets—for the coronavirus project, they had an "open check." Soon after, Reuters got wind of the discussions in New York, breaking the news to the world, and to BioNTech's business development director, Roshni Bhakta.

On the morning after the leak, on Saturday, March 14, a tired Roshni, who had been up until the early hours finalizing an initial term sheet—or internal wish list—jumped on a call with Sean and James Ryan, BioNTech's general counsel, as well as one external lawyer. The quartet were about to have the first of many virtual discussions about the COVID-19 collaboration with their counterparts at Pfizer and needed to make sure they were all on the same page before negotiations began. "You cannot be too intimidated just because they have teams of people behind them," Sean advised Roshni, who had arrived at the company after the influenza vaccine deal with Pfizer had been signed.

For the British executive, this was déjà vu. He had led talks on the proposed flu partnership in 2018 and learned that the U.S. corporation was a force to be reckoned with. He would enter meetings in a London skyscraper flanked by a newly hired James and two lawyers, only to be met by an army of Pfizer representatives, including a senior business development person, a junior business development person, an alliance manager, an IP lawyer, a deal lawyer, an *external* deal lawyer *and* their junior, and a couple of supply chain specialists. "It was a classic David-versus-Goliath situation," Sean remembers. His opposite numbers, all exceedingly well briefed, were not shy about making their demands known.

That first call, in early March, however, "was extraordinary," says Sean, who was astounded by the spirit of cooperation emanating from across the virtual table. The dozen or so negotiators that made up Team Pfizer had been given their orders from on high. "This is the right thing to do," Sean recalls them saying. "Let's get moving."

The first order of business was to put together a so-called letter of intent. BioNTech had already constructed its core COVID-19 vaccine candidates and was testing them on mice to decide which four to take into the clinic. These constructs needed to be sent to Pfizer, pronto, so that the company could start running its own studies in the U.S., both to comply with requirements from the American regulator and to confirm the data from German trials. But there needed to be some basic agreement before the vaccines—the most precious commodity BioNTech had ever produced—could be shipped across the Atlantic and before scientists in Mainz started sharing the underlying science with their new team members.

Over the next three days, Roshni, James, and Sean worked almost around the clock—no longer able to go into the office, as BioNTech had locked down on the Friday that Reuters broke the news of the planned Pfizer partnership—sending drafts of the initial document back and forth every few hours and forwarding them to the U.S. for review.

Meanwhile, the proposed partnership with China's Fosun, which had kept Uğur and Özlem busy during their February holiday in the Canary Islands, was on the brink of being finalized. Unlike with the Pfizer deal, these two companies had barely met before; they had first talked in 2016, and Fosun had briefly considered investing in BioNTech's first funding round, but the discussions hadn't come to anything. Attempting to quickly build a rapport, Ryan had visited the company's representatives on a trip to New York in early February, and soon after, Uğur had gone over to Boston to meet Fosun executive Aimin Hui. "I was very impressed by Uğur," Aimin recalls. "He was an outstanding immunologist, outstanding clinician, and outstanding entrepreneur."

With that relationship cemented, the Fosun deal gathered pace—spearheaded by Ryan and Uğur, without much interference from the business development team at BioNTech. The contract was much more straightforward—this would be, in essence, a licensing deal. There were no concerns about intellectual property or the transfer of technology. Fosun would help BioNTech run clinical trials in China, but the German company would manufacture the vaccines for the country at its European plants and ship them to Asia.

On Monday, March 16, BioNTech announced a "strategic alliance" with Fosun—in which the group would pay up to $135 million for the right to sell the product in China and surrounding territories. The press release also served as public confirmation of the existence of Project Lightspeed. For seven weeks, even as dozens of pharmaceutical companies broadcast their intent to develop coronavirus vaccines far and wide, the scheme had remained under wraps. Now, with the global coronavirus death toll exceeding seven thousand,[10] BioNTech was telling the world that its candidate could be in the clinic by late April, with a pledge to "disclose more in the coming weeks." If Uğur and Özlem's bold bet stumbled, or even failed, there would now be nowhere to hide. The couple, however, felt no added pressure. "We were in full-on focus mode," says Özlem. "We hardly noticed the change."

Roshni had not paused to acknowledge the Fosun news. She was too busy poring over the initial terms for a Pfizer deal—which, by Monday evening, were almost ironed out. "Once in a while, my nine-year-old daughter and I sleep in the living room so we can do like a girls' camp," she says, and it was in that environment, her face lit by the glow of a laptop screen, that she emailed what would become a historic letter to Sierk Poetting, for his signature. At around midnight, it was sent to Pfizer for approval, and the agreement was announced the next morning.

In the space of two days, BioNTech had gone from a largely unknown German business to being part of development and distribution alliances with two enormous pharma groups, with a plan that *could* make a vaccine, if authorized by regulators, available to most of the world. With Pfizer agreeing to let BioNTech defer its share of the costs, amounting to some $190 million, there would also be a massive influx of funds and some breathing room when it came to investments. The news was greeted warmly by the markets. Pharmaceutical analysts at Germany's Berenberg Bank put out a note saying that the company "appears best positioned in the COVID-19 race owing to its diversified mRNA platform, delivery formulation and manufacturing capacity."[11]

Not all the attention was that welcome. With BioNTech's vaccine plans now out in the open, hundreds of letters—some racist, some containing death threats—started arriving at the Mainz campus, where it was left to lab manager François Perrineau to open them. "In the beginning, I had to read these messages," he says. The language used to describe Uğur and Özlem, and the hate directed toward them because of their faith or background, "had an effect on me," he admits.

There was also plenty of abuse that François was unable to intercept. Receptionists at BioNTech were hounded by irate callers. "How does it feel to work for a company that is poisoning the world?" one demanded to know. Then there were the usual suspects who made false claims Uğur and Özlem were working with Bill Gates to insert microchips into unsuspecting patients. Bizarrely, there were also some agitators who seemed to have no concerns about the safety of the vaccine. A handful turned up at BioNTech's front gate, rolled up their sleeves, and demanded to be injected against COVID-19.

François wasted no time in tightening up security. He bought an airport-style scanner to inspect all parcels arriving at headquarters and spoke to the relevant authorities in all the German states where BioNTech had sites, making sure there was a point person the company could call in an emergency. The names of all of BioNTech's suppliers, he ensured, would stay secret for now, unless they chose to volunteer the information themselves. All board members were offered personal protection.

The nascent COVID-19 partnership with Pfizer was fraught with another kind of risk. The day after the letter of intent between the two companies was signed, the collaboration was kicked off with a Zoom call involving roughly sixty managers and scientists from both sides of the Atlantic, to discuss the transfer of BioNTech's closely guarded proprietary technology. "I had told our team: 'Share everything,'" Uğur says, but many of his staff reacted with disbelief, wanting to know exactly what he meant by "everything." "They said, 'Are you sure? These are our holy secrets!'"

A large company, they knew, could simply steal its smaller partner's expertise. In fact, the industry was rife with such allegations. Some Pfizer scientists were researching RNA in California, and while there was no suggestion that the U.S. giant would act in bad faith, it *could* always try to claim that it had independently amassed similar know-how to BioNTech and plow ahead with its own drugs based on the molecule.

But Uğur was adamant. With no time to lose, BioNTech must begin exchanging information with Pfizer, he said, even if a full agreement had not been signed. A virtual data room was soon set up to securely transfer intellectual property. "If this was an ordinary project, there's no way you'd have agreed to this," says Sean. Due to the speed with which it allowed

Pfizer to learn about the vaccine's design, he adds, "it could prove in hindsight to be one of the more critical decisions we've made."

Meanwhile, he and Roshni were racing to formalize the working arrangement with Pfizer. Immediately after signing the letter of intent, "the real work began," Roshni says, and five days later, the two parties exchanged the first draft of a formal contract, which would end up being some two hundred pages long. A redline document—a paper marked-up with amendments and deletions—was sent back and forth between the companies' respective teams every five to seven hours, followed by phone and video calls that lasted an age. "This is what we did every day, including weekends," says Roshni. On one session, she realized she had been on a Zoom conference for over five hours in a row without taking a break. "You start going a bit crazy," she says.

The time difference did not help matters; Pfizer staff were getting up in the early hours in New York, while the BioNTech negotiators in Germany were staying up late. All were starting to flag, and the magnanimity of the initial interactions between the two groups began to fade. "You could tell from the first moment you were on the phone with them that each side was going to be loyal and defend their company to the end," says Roshni. "There was a lot of tension, a lot of anger, but that's because everyone was doing their job completely correctly."

For its part, BioNTech was planning for success, but it also had to prepare for failure. "We had to be realistic and consider a route in which the program didn't make it," says Roshni, "either after spending hundreds and millions of dollars in development, and not achieving market approval, or even a scenario in which we achieve approval but face heavy expenses," such as fees for patented vaccine components. Pfizer agreed to indemnify its prospective partner against such an eventuality, and mechanisms to protect BioNTech from going completely under were added to the contract. But Pfizer sought to use that generosity as leverage as discussions moved from topic to topic, from sharing liability to where each company's name would appear on vials.

The scrimmages did not slow down the process by much. Normally, it would take at least six months to go from drafting a term sheet to closing a deal. The Fosun collaboration—a simpler arrangement—had been finalized in just two months. With Pfizer, an initial agreement was done and dusted on April 9, just twenty-one days after the letter of intent. But it did take a round-the-clock effort. "I think in the final stretch we negotiated for thirty-six hours straight," says Roshni. "I just went from Tuesday night . . . and then we signed it on Thursday morning." There was no celebration, just exhaustion, and relief that the two companies' scientists could now go full speed ahead. Sean sent an email to BioNTech's management and supervisory boards, saying, "It's done."

Seventy-two hours earlier, that outcome had looked less likely. Roshni had been wrestling with her Pfizer peers over the power to have the final say on several key decisions, from selecting the final candidate for clinical trials, to designing such global studies, to deciding on how and where the vaccine should be manufactured. A table was drawn up and each potential conflict argued over in detail. "We had fought tooth and nail," says Roshni, who had thought carefully about how to structure the agreement. The finish line was drawing near, but there were still several sticking points. BioNTech was, after all, a company of 1,300 employees, making demands of a company of 70,000. "They were very polished," says Roshni admiringly of her Pfizer peers, which is something coming from someone intimidatingly put together herself. She kept a tray of makeup next to her computer throughout the process to help her put on a brave face in the endless Zoom calls. But after dozens of hours of intense back-and-forth discussions, negotiations had reached an impasse.

By 11:00 p.m., Roshni was falling asleep at her laptop when Sean called. He had spoken to Uğur, who was dismayed by the delay. "It just has to work," Uğur had told him, referring to the agreement. "I do not want business development or legal to get in the way of the science."

To resolve the situation, yet another call was set up between the two negotiating teams. This time, however, Kathrin Jansen joined, as did Uğur. "We start talking and going through the table," says Roshni, "and

Uğur interrupts us." What he said next sent her and Sean's jaws to the floor. "Each company should focus on their strengths," Uğur calmly insisted. BioNTech should take the lead on matters of mRNA technology and clinical studies in Europe, "and we should decide on these topics." But when it came to other matters, such as the Phase 3 trial, it should either be solely Pfizer's decision or a joint one. Even the authorization rights BioNTech had already won during the negotiations, he said, should revert to being mutual ones, if necessary. "Luckily, I wasn't on-screen," says Roshni, "because, I was like, 'F**k.'" Step by step, her boss was unraveling everything the trio had been fighting for. Sean was frantically texting Uğur: "Stop talking, we have final say!" But he went on in the same vein for another twenty minutes. "This development won't happen," Uğur told his staff in front of the whole meeting, "if we don't let the other party do their work."

Reflecting on that moment more than a year later, Roshni acknowledges that she and Sean were thinking with their business and legal hats on—"How much can we grab and hold?"—while Uğur saw the situation purely in terms of "How can we make decisions efficiently and get this thing done?" Every impediment to progress in the agreement was ripped up, including the arbitration mechanism, by which, if a decision could not be reached within thirty days, parties had the right to take the matter to court. "Uğur said, 'Just get rid of all that,'" Roshni, who is still astounded by the move, remembers. "He said, 'If we wait for arbitration, we'll never address the pandemic.'"

Uğur and Özlem had suffered from relinquishing sovereignty before and had spent years fiercely protecting their hard-fought independence. Thanks to the patience and deep pockets of the Strüngmann brothers, they had clung to their self-governance for more than a decade. Now, for the biggest undertaking of their lives, they would be placing their trust in Big Pharma. At every stage of Project Lightspeed, no one would leave the virtual room until a joint decision was reached.

FIRST IN HUMAN

It was the combination of Kate Winslet, Matt Damon, and Jude Law that first got Claudia Lindemann thinking about public health crises. One evening in 2011, while studying for her master's in pharmaceutical science in Münster, Germany, she had watched the movie *Contagion*. Inspired by the first SARS outbreak, in which the world is brought to a standstill by a previously unknown pathogen, the film is eerily prescient. Although she found the lab scenes "unrealistic," Claudia, an amateur actor herself, couldn't help but wonder "what it takes to develop a vaccine in a pandemic." Little did she know that nine years later, she would find herself thrust into a central, real-life role.

In the meeting on February 6, weeks before Pfizer and Fosun came on board the Lightspeed train, Germany's Paul Ehrlich Institute had rejected BioNTech's appeal for a so-called toxicology study to be run simultaneously with clinical trials or skipped altogether. Before a "first in human"—or Phase 1 trial—could begin, the regulator had insisted, rats injected with the mRNA constructs would need to be observed for signs of serious side effects over several weeks. Their organ tissues would have to be examined under a microscope for signs of disease and the resulting data compiled in a formally verified report. Thankfully, this time-consuming task was one for which Claudia was well prepared.

After finishing her master's degree, she had become one of the first beneficiaries of the European VacTrain initiative, set up to nurture a new generation of vaccine developers, and had done her doctorate on the topic at Oxford's prestigious Jenner Institute (where, unbeknownst to Claudia, her former colleagues were already working on their own coronavirus vaccine). In 2018, she was hired by BioNTech and, as a trained virologist with no cancer expertise to speak of, was put in charge of running the toxicology study for the flu vaccine collaboration with Pfizer. This six-month process had just begun when Claudia was told of the coronavirus project and the PEI's request.

This time, she knew, "the tox" would have to be completed *much* faster. In a discussion with Uğur soon after that February meeting with the regulator, Claudia explained that she had worked on condensing every step of the study and had managed to reduce its duration to just three months. Uğur was less impressed than she had hoped. He wanted to start clinical trials within weeks. "Come on, Claudia," he said, "we need to find a solution."

In search of such a solution, Claudia returned to her desk in one of BioNTech's satellite offices—situated above an old brewery in Mainz's medieval center. There, she clicked on a report she had come across a few days earlier, after googling "How do you develop a vaccine in a pandemic?"

The 113-page paper, entitled "Guidelines on the Quality, Safety and Efficacy of Ebola Vaccines,"[1] had been drafted more than three years earlier by an expert committee at the World Health Organization and was primarily concerned with the vaccines developed in the wake of the epidemic in West Africa. But it also contained some general principles for drugmakers rushing to contain *any* rampant virus. With Uğur's words ringing in her ears, Claudia set about looking for ways to speed the study up.

Buried on page 55, she found a crucial passage. The phrasing was impenetrable for nonexperts, but the authors were essentially advising regulators that in a public health emergency, drug developers should be allowed to proceed to a Phase 1 trial after compiling an *interim* report. It would contain data gathered from the observation of the rodents and from blood tests taken soon after the vaccines were administered, to show that the substance had not severely harmed rats. But the most time-consuming part of a toxicology study—the part in which the rats' organs are carefully dissected and the samples scrutinized under microscopes—would not have to be completed for a human trial to begin. If the furry subjects were found to be healthy soon after being injected, BioNTech would be able to start its Phase 1 trial immediately and complete the rest of the toxicology study while the clinical trial was ongoing.

Claudia presented this proposal in virtual meetings with the regulator, and the Paul Ehrlich experts gave her plan the go-ahead.

The analysis phase, however, was not the only hurdle in the way of a speedy tox. Regulations required companies to administer one *extra* dose in animal studies than the number planned for human trials.

To disrupt the docking mechanism by which the SARS-CoV-2 spike protein—that crown-like protrusion—attaches to specific receptors and invades healthy cells, BioNTech and most other vaccine developers had opted for a two-shot regimen. "If you don't know the power of the enemy, you don't want the response to be too weak," Uğur had told the team in early meetings, much to the disappointment of commercially minded managers who were hoping for an easy-to-sell, one-shot product. When first exposed to a perceived threat, he explained, the immune system produces a so-called prime response. Upon the second encounter, the body's defenses are boosted. "We don't know what is needed," Uğur said, "so let's go for the maximum."

Hearing this, Claudia had done the math. Two doses in clinical trials would mean that she would have to test *three* consecutive doses in rats. Since the Lightspeed team had decided to leave twenty-one days—or three weeks—between each injection in humans, the dosing of rodents in the toxicology study would take six weeks and only after that period was up would final blood samples be analyzed. Uğur's goal was unachievable.

Stumped, she returned to the drawing board. Claudia soon concluded that the only remaining option was to shorten the three-week intervals. BioNTech would dose the rodents three times, but only a week apart. This, she argued to the PEI experts, was an even more intense protocol—if the animals tolerated being repeatedly given that much vaccine, one could assume that humans would fare fine with greater gaps between administrations.

The design, however, posed a risk to Project Lightspeed's ambitious timelines. BioNTech planned to inject one group of rodents with the highest dose it intended to use in clinical trials—100 micrograms. This was a lot of vaccine for an animal weighing between 200 and 300 grams, and it would probably cause some temporary side effects, including swelling. Due to the condensed recovery period, such symptoms, which would normally subside in time, might appear more serious than they actually were and be mistaken for a problematic adverse event.

Claudia, however, was confident. She remembered the BCG vaccine against meningitis and tuberculosis that she had been given as a kid, which left a large sore. "I did not think we would have local reactogenicity worse than that," she says, "so I advocated, even in front of the PEI, that local tolerances are no issue." If she was right, her bold move would help furnish BioNTech with enough animal safety data to apply for the launch of a first-in-human clinical trial just three weeks after dosing the first rats in a toxicology study.

With this innovative design in place, Claudia roared into action alongside Jan Diekmann, a former member of Uğur and Özlem's academic group in Mainz, who now led BioNTech's nonclinical safety department. They ordered rats to be sent to a certified testing site as soon as possible to give the animals time to acclimatize. They made sure the mRNA material for the study was sent to Polymun in Austria and, once formulated, driven to the facility that was housing the study. But someone needed to be there to supervise the start of the tox on Tuesday, March 17.

On the day before the planned kickoff, Angela Merkel took to a stage in Berlin. The number of coronavirus deaths in Germany had risen to sixteen, and confirmed cases had jumped by a fifth in just twenty-four hours, to over six thousand. Three days after Sierk had sent everyone but essential BioNTech staff home, the chancellor implored citizens to cancel their holidays and stay at home wherever possible. Churches and synagogues should close, she said, as well as playgrounds and nonessential shops. "There have never been measures like this in our country before," Merkel told a press conference. "They are far-reaching, but at the moment, they are necessary."[2] Claudia was moving home, and with kindergartens now closed, she had a small child in need of constant care and attention. There was no way she could travel. So, on Monday afternoon, Jan got into his Mercedes and began the long drive to the toxicology site, in south Germany.

As he was speeding down the uncannily empty autobahn, Jan's phone rang. It was Claudia, with a strange request. The plan for the toxicology study, in which every detail of the design was written down—from precise dosages to intervals, to when blood samples were to be drawn—had been signed off by all parties. But while she was confident that most of the coronavirus vaccine candidates—being administered in three different dose sizes—would be well tolerated in rats, Claudia suddenly had some concerns about one of the constructs—based on uRNA. The maximum dose of 100 micrograms "may be too high," she said. Annette Vogel's team was already injecting the construct in mice at BioNTech, to test for antibodies. They had observed that the rodents were losing weight, which was a clear indication of intolerability. "I really don't feel good about this," Claudia told Jan. "Let's request an amendment to the plan."

With the rats set to be dosed at 8:00 a.m. the following day, this request was a highly unusual one. Jan had to work quickly, and immediately sent an email to the tox study organizers.

At 7:00 the next morning, the plan was amended and sent back to BioNTech for signing. Meanwhile, Jan drove from his hotel to an old farmhouse that had been converted into the animal testing facility. He disinfected his hands, put on protective clothing, and headed into the room in which individually numbered rats were being weighed and having their temperature taken. But in one corner of the barn, employees were injecting the 100-microgram dose of uRNA that had caused Claudia to fret. "The workers were so eager to start that they had already dosed two animals before the message to abort came through," she says.

The rodents were taken out of the official study, but Jan decided to have them monitored in any case. Perhaps, he thought, they would provide a useful clue as to how well this platform was tolerated in high doses.

As Claudia and Jan worked on a Lightspeed toxicology study, others at BioNTech were grappling with the task of launching the fastest first-in-human trial in its history.

The company had plenty of experience in administering mRNA pharmaceuticals to cancer patients and had dosed more than four hundred people over the years across several clinical trials and countries. Such studies, however, were slow-moving affairs. Hospitals around the world were contracted to identify people at a specific stage of advanced disease who were willing to take an experimental drug. Recruiting the required number of patients took years.

Designing a Phase 1 for a coronavirus vaccine, by contrast, *should* have been a walk in the park. BioNTech would be able to draw from healthy volunteers across society and merely needed to monitor for side effects, which the participants would log in diaries and reveal in phone conversations with investigators. On the day the German contractor that was to run the trial for the COVID-19 candidates put out a call for volunteers on Facebook,[3] more than a thousand people came forward in a single day. Some even called BioNTech's front desk and begged to be included. Finding willing subjects was not going to be a challenge.

There were, however, plenty of hurdles to navigate.

For a start, the company did not even have enough staff to prepare such studies for its existing oncology pipeline. On that fateful weekend in January, Özlem had been sifting through résumés to expand the team of medical directors and clinical developers at BioNTech. As Project Lightspeed kicked into gear, those applicants were still being interviewed.

Because the compounds of the coronavirus vaccine had never been tested on humans, this would also be a complex trial. Volunteers would

first receive very low doses of the vaccine, and only if that was well tolerated would a higher dose be given to other participants. As Uğur and
Özlem planned to take a handful of the twenty candidates they were currently testing into the clinic, the trial would need to assess the safety and
tolerability of each construct at escalating doses, in different age groups,
before the best candidate and the right dose could be chosen for a combined Phase 2 and 3 trial run by Pfizer, involving tens of thousands of
subjects.

The German contractor running the Phase 1 would have to adapt its
normal working processes to enable an unusually efficient study. Like
most companies in the country, however, it did not operate on weekends.
It was by no means a given that the team would come in on Saturdays
and Sundays, even for such a critical project. The dosing schedule had to
be planned carefully so that key dates for reviewing data from blood tests
did not land on weekends.

Then there was the matter of communication and training. Handing a
new pharmaceutical into the care of clinicians to conduct a clinical trial
is a little like leaving an infant with a babysitter for the first time. A parent will leave detailed instructions explaining when the child needs to
be fed, how often she cries, and how to calm her. Similarly, to make sure
a human study is not paused at the first sign of a side effect, regulators,
and those staffing the trial, need to be told exactly which symptoms are
within the realm of the expected and how to gauge the risk they pose to
patients. To this end, the company needed to quickly create an investigators' brochure, essentially a user manual containing a rundown of the
technology behind the vaccines. Its purpose was to eliminate surprises.

It was the middle of March, and until now, the cutting-edge science
behind Project Lightspeed had only been imparted to experts in the field,
including Klaus Cichutek and the PEI panel, contract manufacturers,
as well as staff at BioNTech, Fosun, and Pfizer. This brochure would be
the first attempt to comprehensively explain how the vaccine candidates
worked to outsiders. It would need to be a crash course in language that
a physician who has never so much as seen a strand of mRNA could understand.

There was no one at BioNTech who had the knowledge and expertise to bring all of this together. No one, that is, except Özlem.

Her unique skills were already a crucial component of the couple's personal and professional partnership. Were it left up to Uğur—a visual thinker—he would cover the walls of his office with whiteboards and notes. Each of these mind maps made sense to him, of course, and may even have made sense to experts in particular fields. But someone needed to draw a coherent thread between them, to connect the dots. "We needed to explain things to nonspecialists," says Özlem. She honed this skill as the pair moved into translational medicine, bringing their innovations from the lab directly to patients' bedsides.

The same was true of BioNTech's 120-odd research projects. Both Uğur and Özlem understood the sum of the parts, the overarching vision, but only she could communicate this to others. "I start with the pieces, and she starts with the integrated view," says Uğur admiringly. It was, therefore, Özlem who crafted the narrative of BioNTech's mRNA vaccines and therapies. It was Özlem who presented the company's breakthroughs—where possible in immaculate German—to conferences, colleges, and capital markets. It was Özlem who became, in Uğur's words, "the integrator, the translator, the closer."

At BioNTech's—and humankind's—hour of need, these talents came in handy. As the company's chief medical officer, Özlem made sure that the investigators in the proposed Phase 1 trial understood the potential for fever and flu-like symptoms and that it was perfectly fine to use anti-inflammatory drugs to treat them. She compiled a list of easy-to-read tips, including the suggestion, for example, that volunteers be well hydrated before receiving their injections. But that was just the routine stuff.

Together with Martin Bexon, an external medical consultant, and Christopher Marshallsay, BioNTech's head of medical writing, Özlem also took on the task of designing and crafting the study protocol, in which the entire structure of the clinical trial needed to be outlined. Before doing that, however, she had to negotiate with the Paul Ehrlich Institute and a separate Ethics Commission on how to enable a quick selection of a final Phase 3 vaccine candidate.

Normally, the single ascending dose process described earlier would take months to complete—months BioNTech did not have. During initial discussions with Pfizer's clinical colleagues, it became clear that it was imperative that the final-stage trial begin by the end of July to have an approved vaccine in 2020. But Özlem realized that even if the BioNTech Phase 1 trial started in April and was conducted perfectly in the minimum possible time, it would not be over before September. Something had to give.

Discussions with the regulators went back and forth on how many "sentinels"—volunteers who receive the first doses—were required and how long they needed to be monitored before others could be injected with the same dose size. There were deliberations over what data would be required from those who received a lower dose, for the trial to be able to move to the next step, with some participants getting a higher dose. Özlem argued that safety data from BioNTech's mRNA oncology trials and early data from Claudia's toxicology study had shown that most adverse events were observed within the first twenty-four hours of administration. She proposed that a portion of the remaining participants in each twelve-person group could therefore be jabbed just a day after the sentinel. The rest would follow forty-eight hours later, to further mitigate risk.

Özlem and her team also identified another way to accelerate the trial. In a non-pandemic situation, most clinical studies would be designed so that the second shot was given after an interval of at least twenty-eight days to give the immune response prompted by the first shot more time to get going. After the double dosing was complete, investigators would wait for fourteen more days before they checked for the existence of antibodies and T-cells. It would therefore take forty-two days before blood samples could even be collected. For the COVID-19 trials, Özlem and her team decided to implement a vaccination schedule with a gap of just twenty-one days and test for immune responses seven days after the second shot, rather than two weeks. In total, this would shave fourteen days off the entire process.

That fortnight would not only help a Phase 3 trial launch on time. Months later, it would also ensure that people receiving the vaccine in the real world got their second shots sooner—after twenty-one days, rather than twenty-eight—and were therefore fully protected faster.

After reviewing the data, the authorities agreed to both these concepts, significantly reducing the time it would take to complete a first-in-human study.

BioNTech shared the clinical trial plan with Pfizer so that the American company could run a similar process in the U.S. Not only would the repeated trial serve to mollify the FDA, which preferred drug developers to run a domestic version of such studies, but it would also, hopefully, confirm the data gathered in Mannheim and at another site in Berlin.

After three weeks of lockdown, data released by Germany's health agency, the Robert Koch Institute, showed that the worst-case scenario Uğur had envisioned in January—of rapid, uncontrollable spread of SARS-CoV-2—had not been realized. Instead, basic containment measures were controlling the virus, giving BioNTech some breathing room. For three months, he and Özlem had lived on the edge. Now they were more confident that with the accelerated toxicology study and innovative first-in-human trial in place, science might just outpace this pathogen. "I knew we had a chance," says Uğur. "We were in the game."

Still, the Lightspeed team needed to reduce complexity. Quickly. Most manufacturers had selected a single, ideal candidate to take to the clinic. Moderna had done that on March 16, when it dosed the first patient with its mRNA vaccine, designed to express the full spike protein that protrudes from the coronavirus. Scientists at Oxford University, who would later team up with AstraZeneca, chose to assess a lone make-or-break viral vector construct too.

There was no way that BioNTech's twenty constructs—each with a different genetic code for the spike protein or based on a different mRNA platform—could all be tested on humans, in escalating doses, while sticking to an ambitious timeline. When it came to a Phase 1 clinical trial, the company would need to whittle down its candidates.

In the labs that lined the upper floors of BioNTech's Mainz HQ, the Lightspeed team were doing their bit to narrow down the selection.

It was too early to get results from Claudia's toxicology study or an indication of the T-cells the candidates were able to prompt. But since that first visualization—the graph Uğur used as a screen saver—had shown that the vaccines were capable of inducing an immune response in mice, a slew of similar data had trickled in. It showed that all twenty preclinical prototypes prompted the development of strong neutralizing antibodies. There was not much to choose between them.

The team knew, however, that while readouts from rodent studies are *indicative,* the data was not necessarily *predictive* of how a vaccine would work in humans. As a hedge against this potential disparity, Özlem says, "we wanted to test at least one construct per mRNA platform in the Phase 1," referring to the proprietary formats in BioNTech's toolbox, and to have an equal split between candidates coding for the spike protein itself and the smaller receptor-binding domain. Even in an accelerated first-in-human trial, the company wanted as many shots on goal as possible.

The key, in Uğur's and Özlem's minds, was to find a vaccine that achieved the right balance between two essential features. One was to ensure that the protein for which the mRNA encoded—the target used to train troops—was reproduced in cells in large numbers. The other was to stimulate the immune system. Too little stimulation, and a reasonable dose of mRNA could fail to activate all relevant forces, such as antibodies and T-cells. Too much could result in serious side effects.

The first platform included by the couple, uRNA, was naturally endowed with the ability to trigger immune activity, and, as proven by the treatment of hundreds of cancer patients, the BioNTech team had achieved great results with the format when wrapped in a neutral lipid for intravenous administration. But the uRNA had never been combined with the new lipids being proposed for intramuscular injection, which had their own, complementary stimulatory powers. There was a risk that together, this formulation would overwhelm the immune system. To avoid this, the team could have subjected the uRNA to a particular purification process developed by BioNTech, but Uğur did not want to add even more complexity. BioNTech would just have to test the uRNA in its unpurified form and hope for the best.

The modRNA, conversely, which had been originally developed for an entirely different purpose, blunted stimulatory activity. Therefore, Uğur says, although "we knew that modRNA would be well tolerated, we were worried that the T-cell response might not be as strong as that achieved with uRNA and that the dose needed might be in the range of 200–300 micrograms (that's up to ten times higher than the dose of the vaccine that eventually made it to market)." The lipids' ability to trigger immune activity, which could compromise the uRNA candidates, might, in contrast, help the modRNA. The only way to find out was to put both in the study. A single uRNA-based candidate and two modRNA-based candidates—one encoding for the full spike and one for the receptor-binding domain—were selected for clinical testing.

The final slot was given to the youngest of all the platforms, the self-amplifying, or saRNA, for a vaccine encoding for the full spike, taking the number of first-in-human candidates to a process-stretching maximum of four. But while both uRNA and modRNA had gone through multiple adjustments by the BioNTech team over the years, saRNA had not been refined in such a manner. It had not passed the preclinical antibody tests with flying colors. Nonetheless, because the platform caused mRNA to reproduce itself for a short while after injection, the saRNA came with the promise of lower doses, and Uğur decided to give it a shot as a contingency plan. The new kid on the block might also form the basis of a second-generation vaccine, he thought, if results from the Phase 1 trial helped the company to tweak the saRNA's formula.

Information about the selected candidates was passed on to the manufacturing team in Idar-Oberstein, the site outside where the train had been stopped in February, panicking Sierk into introducing tougher restrictions at BioNTech. This was no dummy run—vaccines produced for clinical trials had to adhere to extremely high standards, to avoid contamination or dud formulations, and required intensive preparation. BioNTech's DNA template and RNA manufacturing teams worked in shifts to compile detailed instructions for every step of the process.

For each candidate, the DNA had to be produced first as a template to produce the mRNA. The steps took a total of five days—from Monday to Friday. To allow staff some rest over the weekend—after working for days on end in clean rooms, clad from head to toe in stuffy hazmat suits, pausing only every few hours for food and toilet breaks—one production run was scheduled per week. The mRNA for the modRNA candidate encoding for the receptor-binding domain was produced first, followed by the unmodified version. As with the first test batches produced after Stephanie's cloning team overcame their initial difficulties to "play like world champions," a small, white panel van waited outside the BioNTech plant to drive the mRNA material, packed in plastic bags and frozen at minus 70 degrees Celsius, overnight to Polymun in Vienna. There, it was combined with lipids before being bottled, labeled, and sent to clinical trial sites.

By the afternoon of Thursday, April 16, BioNTech was ready for its first-in-human study to begin. With four candidates chosen and production schedules in place, the company was about to submit an official application for a Phase 1 trial to the Paul Ehrlich Institute. Then, an email arrived in Uğur's and Özlem's inboxes. Alex Muik, who had been testing for neutralizing antibodies as fast as his single tabletop machine would let him, had attached new data on yet *another* construct, based on modRNA and expressing the full spike protein. The nucleotide sequence for the knobby prong had been slightly tweaked to optimize how it was translated by cells in the body. The vaccine, called BNT162b2.9, had only recently been tested in mice, and blood from the rodents had just been drawn and delivered to Alex. But the results were clear: it had prompted a *far* superior antibody response to the similar modRNA construct, BNT162b2.8, that had already been selected as a candidate.

Uğur immediately picked up his smartphone and called Alex, then Annette Vogel, to get more details. Both agreed that the B2.9 would be a better finalist and were disappointed that it was too late to include in the human study, which was due to start within days. Uğur, however, was not ready to give up. "Let's see what we can do here," he told the duo before hanging up and calling Andreas Kuhn, who was overseeing the manu-facturing in Idar-Oberstein.

"We can't change the construct and have it ready on Monday," came the response when Uğur asked for the impossible. "Not even at the speed of light." The production process took five days, Andreas reminded Uğur, and in any case, the next week's capacity was already earmarked for pro-ducing the B2.8 candidate for the clinical trial. Uğur paused for a few seconds, leaving Andreas to wonder if the line had gone dead. What if, he mused, the team brought forward the production of the self-amplifying construct by a week, reversing the order of the dosing in the clinical trial, and giving BioNTech time to prepare a switch to the B2.9? The team, An-dreas replied, had worked tirelessly to prepare all the documents for the older version, "but I'll talk to them." On Friday evening, he called back. The Idar-Oberstein staff, who had just completed a grueling five-day stint, would work through the weekend to prepare an alternative production run. Uğur sent a single-line email to Alex and Annette: "We'll make B2.9 work." Nine months later, it would become abundantly clear how signif-icant this decision was in finally curbing the spread of the coronavirus.

Claudia, meanwhile, was putting the finishing touches on a nine-hundred-page interim report from her toxicology study, which had taken just two months.

The data was remarkably good. The rats did not develop a high fever or lose weight. There were no warning signs, such as rough fur, which can in-dicate that the animals are out of sorts. The rodents also scurried away when investigators entered the room, as they are instinctively prone to do when healthy. "If they just sit in the corner and don't do anything, that's bad," says Claudia, "but they were just perfectly happy." There was no inkling of a severe systemic response to any of the selected mRNA vaccine candidates. The mammalian immune system was not being overloaded.

However, Claudia's gut feeling on that afternoon before the study began, when she called Jan in his Mercedes and asked for the 100-microgram doses of uRNA to be removed at the last minute, had proved to be prophetic. The two rodents injected with that highest dose by overeager technicians—before the instructions to abort came through—developed a fever of over 40 degrees Celsius. Thankfully, the rats had been taken out of the study before it began, so the data would not hold up approval of the clinical trial.

But after BioNTech submitted the clean toxicology data to the PEI, on April 16, the regulator realized that the candidates selected for the first-in-human study were not all identical to the ones Claudia and Jan had tested on rats. The B2.9, which had been subbed on by Uğur at the very last minute, had, of course, not been a part of the rodent toxicology study that had started back in March.

Claudia was cold-called by experts at the agency who demanded an explanation. With her smartphone running out of battery life and her young child in the other room, she was forced to kneel down near a plug socket and speak to the PEI while her phone was charging. From this position, she reiterated that BioNTech was running a study with a so-called platform approach, following guidance found in another part of the WHO's Ebola report. A closely related candidate, B2.8, had been tested in the tox study and could be considered to be a proxy for the B2.9, which was based on the exact same platform in the BioNTech mRNA toolbox. They belonged to the same family.

BioNTech and Pfizer would soon test the B2.9 in rats too, she assured the regulator, but not in time for the start of human studies in Mannheim and Berlin. "We said the exact candidate is still coming," says Jan, who joined the call, "and we have no doubt that the results will be comparable."

There was, however, one final bureaucratic hurdle. At the end of March, while in discussions with Özlem and her team, the Ethics Commission in the state of Baden-Württemberg had decreed that all trial participants would have to be tested for COVID-19 before they were administered a vaccine. At the time, only a few specialist companies were able to test for the disease, and it took at least a couple of days to process the results. Even the topflight Bundesliga football league, which had been suspended for weeks, was struggling to get its players tested regularly enough to safely resume matches. In so many other ways, the Ethics Commission had been extremely supportive—scheduling ad hoc meetings with the team and with regulators—so the sudden requirement came as a surprise. "It was difficult to understand," says Uğur. "When it came to this topic, we didn't manage to change their minds."

After his protestations proved fruitless, Uğur turned to Christian Miculka, a project manager who had only joined BioNTech in February, for help. Christian immediately called a friend with whom he had studied in Austria thirty years earlier, and who was now working for a former subsidiary of the German company Bosch. The well-known appliances manufacturer, Christian knew, also produced the so-called PCR equipment used for gold standard COVID-19 tests, and so he asked for a contact at the company. Hours later, as he was having his car tires changed in the pouring rain, Christian received a call from a vice president at Bosch. The testing devices were in extraordinarily high demand, he was told, and would cost roughly €50,000 each. Even if enough of the scarce machines could be sourced for BioNTech, the executive said, the disposable cartridges needed for tests to be carried out were a hot commodity and would be extremely difficult to get hold of. Nonetheless, after checking that the equipment met the standards of the Ethics Commission, Christian ordered four of the precious devices and as many cartridges as he could source. "I had to apologize to our procurement team," he says, "as I probably violated all their policies." There had been no time to shop around.

Uğur and Özlem were at home when the email came through, just before 3:00 p.m. on Tuesday, April 21. "PEI: study can start," read the subject line of the message forwarded by BioNTech's regulatory affairs whizz, Ruben Rizzi. A formal response from the German agency was pasted within. "The certificates and test results are appropriate and thus fulfill the respective requirements as laid down in the clinical trial approval," it said. Above the message, Ruben, an energetic Italian whose father—an infectious disease specialist—was seeing to acute COVID-19 patients at an overloaded hospital in Bergamo, added, in block capital letters: "CONGRATULATIONS, EVERYONE."

Hours later, another team member replied-all with a further update. The Bosch PCR machines had arrived at the main clinical trial site in Mannheim. BioNTech employees, who had been studying the manuals for the machines, were traveling to the locations to train those working there. A clinical trial involving two hundred healthy volunteers between eighteen and fifty-five years old would be starting on Uğur's schedule, in April, with older subjects included twenty-eight days after the younger cohort had been dosed twice and monitored. Uğur sent this information to his Pfizer counterparts, adding, "We are still on time."

The news was greeted with some relief in New York, which was fast becoming the global center of the coronavirus pandemic. Intensive care units were overflowing, and the sound of sirens provided an apocalyptic soundtrack for those working on Lightspeed in Pfizer's Manhattan skyscraper. Dozens of mobile morgues were set up in the city, with refrigerated trucks parked outside hospitals[4] to store the dead. Some hospitals ran out of body bags, and unclaimed corpses were being buried in mass graves in a potter's field on Hart Island.[5] "It's one thing if you see a picture on television, it is another thing when you walk through the streets of New York and you see those refrigerator trucks piling up," says Pfizer's Kathrin Jansen.[6] "That was so chilling."

The next day, April 22, the Paul Ehrlich Institute publicly announced[7] that it had authorized BioNTech's clinical trial. Claudia, who had not been among those who received Ruben Rizzi's email, first heard the news from the coronavirus news ticker on Tagesschau, the German public broadcaster's website. An email went out to BioNTech staff soon after, and the company's shares rose by a whopping 30 percent on the Nasdaq in New York. The PEI's leader, Klaus Cichutek, held a press conference in which he ran through the regulator's work in the run-up to the authorization, emphasizing that no corners had been cut. But when asked when a vaccine would be approved for wider use, he dampened expectations. It was "unlikely," he said, before the end of the year.

That same afternoon, fresh data came through on the B2.9 construct, which had been included in the clinical trial at the last minute. It had been a week since the last blood tests of the mice injected with this tweaked construct, and the new samples confirmed that the level of neutralizing antibodies was more than four times higher than those prompted by the B2.8. A relieved Uğur emailed Alex: "Your studies confirm that it *was* a very wise decision to change," he wrote. "Many thanks."

On Thursday, April 23, BioNTech's comms chief, Jasmina Alatovic, headed to the site of the clinical trial in Mannheim, to coordinate filming of the historic moment—the first injection—for the German press. A colleague who was driving down offered Jasmina a lift and asked if she could wait at Frankfurt's airport, which was along the route. The main terminal of this global hub, usually teeming with bankers and holidaymakers, was empty, and the rapid clicking of a retro, flapping departures board was the only sound. Just a couple of taxis were parked in the cab rank outside. A vaccine could not come soon enough.

Once she arrived at the nondescript, brown brick building in Mannheim, events unfolded quickly. As trams trundled by outside, the BioNTech team waited in a small room to protect the anonymity of the volunteers. Next door, a clinician diluted the vaccine, and at 11:08 a.m., the first patient was dosed with the uRNA construct. A one-line message was sent to the Lightspeed team. "The preparation of the vaccine and the injection went smoothly," it read. Within minutes, Özlem had replied-all: "Great job, everybody! I am so proud of all of you, and I find it amazing how this team is able to perform 'high-endurance athlete' style."

Pictures of the moment were broadcast on rolling news channels across the country. A few hours later, the Oxford team would inject its first patient in the UK[8] with a viral vector coronavirus vaccine candidate.

Thanks to the Germans' love of early starts, however, BioNTech became the first company in Europe to test a COVID-19 vaccine in humans.

With the first Phase 1 volunteers safely dosed, the Lightspeed team began the agonizing wait for the first signs of a working vaccine in humans. It was a wait that Özlem and the clinical team's decisions had reduced to five weeks: three weeks until the second dose could be administered, one week for immune defenses to kick in, and one week for the processing of samples. All of a sudden, however, that final processing stage seemed too ambitious.

By this point, BioNTech was using the diagnostics company in northern Italy to analyze samples from the trial. Test tubes from the research centers in Mannheim and Berlin were being couriered directly to the Tuscan firm, now open and running at full capacity. At Uğur's urging, BioNTech was pushing for initial results, in their raw form, to be made available as soon as possible, so that a decision could be made on the winning vaccine candidate for a global final-stage study.

Soon, however, it became clear that the procedure in Italy would take too long. Staff were not working around the clock and, by regulatory decree, had to proofread and double-check data before delivering their conclusions. Once again, Uğur leaned on Alex Muik's resourcefulness. As soon as blood was drawn from double-dosed German trial volunteers, cartons containing the samples were sent to BioNTech. Using the surrogate virus test Alex had worked on, along with his single tabletop machine, preliminary data on whether the vaccines were prompting a strong immune response could be produced within a day. "I kept calling Alex," says Uğur, who was desperate to know how the candidates were faring almost as soon as they had arrived in Mainz. "He would say: 'Uğur, give me three hours,' then 'Uğur, I still need thirty minutes.'" Then, on May 29, just after 1:00 p.m., an email came through.

In it, Alex had attached the very first data set from BioNTech's clinical trial. He had tested the blood of six participants dosed twice with 10 micrograms of the modRNA and two subjects dosed with 30 micrograms of the same formulation—the platform over which Uğur and Özlem had fretted, wondering if it would require an enormous dose. The neutralizing antibodies were measured against sera from recovered COVID-19 patients and represented by a few dozen dots clustered together at the bottom of a what, to the uninitiated, would appear to be an unremarkable plot graph. What the image signified, however, was a monumental advance in science's battle to beat the deadly coronavirus. The candidate was bringing the sharpshooters of the immune system out in force, just seven days after a low-dose regimen was completed—an even better response than that observed in patients who had survived a natural coronavirus infection.

The results were a relief to the Lightspeed team. Eleven days earlier, Moderna had published a readout from four volunteers in its modRNA Phase 1 study. The U.S. biotech had tested a 25-microgram dose, but found it wanting, and said it was moving forward with 50-microgram and 100-microgram doses instead.[9] BioNTech had been desperate to avoid a similar fate, because reports from participants in its German trial who had received 100 micrograms of the modRNA did not make for good reading. The subjects developed flu-like symptoms, including chills and fever. Some could not get out of bed. For a vaccine that was supposed to be administered at record speed, in all sorts of makeshift environments, this was less than ideal. Those getting the shot would have to be closely monitored for hours, and many would no doubt choose to give such an experience a miss. "You ideally want something you can inject in a supermarket car park," says Özlem, who was on the four-person committee that reviewed the safety data from Berlin and Mannheim.

The panel had decided not to continue with 100-microgram doses. But the preliminary data Alex had sent over showed that choice to be inconsequential to the emergence of a working candidate. Quite the contrary. "At that moment, we knew that 10 micrograms, maybe 30 micrograms, might be sufficient," says Uğur. All the mRNA optimizations the couple and their teams had worked on over the years were paying off. "The number of doses we would be able to provide in the event of market authorization had effectively tripled."

Even more encouragingly, the BioNTech modRNA candidate was

activating neutralizing antibodies with similar levels of success in all eight volunteers whose blood had been analyzed. There was a high likelihood that the troops deployed by the body in response to the vaccine would disrupt the pathogen that had already claimed almost half a million lives, preventing it from latching on to lung cells and causing severe disease. "It was wonderful to see," says Uğur, who for a second allowed himself to revel in the beauty of the science he, Özlem, and their teams had spent decades perfecting.

Seven minutes later, he replied to the email. "Dear Alexander, dear team," his response read. "This is incredible. We have a vaccine!"

ON OUR OWN

For many of BioNTech's staff, the emergence of a vaccine that prompted strong immune responses felt like the last mile of a marathon. Sure, there was a global clinical trial still to be run, and supply deals to be agreed, and an enormous logistical challenge to consider. But the pivotal first stage of Project Lightspeed, the hard science, was almost over. They had toiled for months to build twenty candidates, under the most trying circumstances, and pitted them against each other until, in a beautiful epistemological exhibition, at least one of their shots at goal—the modRNA encoding for the receptor-binding domain—looked on target. Whether it would prevent disease in patients infected with COVID-19 in the real world remained unknown, but that was in the hands of the gods.

For Andreas Kuhn, however, the hardest work still lay ahead. One of a handful of core BioNTech employees who had been by Uğur and Özlem's side since the company's inception (he had joined the couple after finding the cutthroat nature of tenure-track academia too much to bear), the silver-haired biochemist had become the resident master of all things manufacturing. Since the start of February 2020, he had overseen the production of COVID-19 vaccine candidates at BioNTech's mRNA production facilities, first in Idar-Oberstein, then in Mainz. His team had generated *just* enough vaccine material to support lab and animal tests and provided the few hundred doses needed for the German Phase 1 trial. But a large-scale study was looming, involving tens of thousands of people around the world, and while BioNTech's technical development experts, led by Ulrich Blaschke, were training Pfizer in the art of mRNA production, it would take months before the pharma giant was ready to manufacture vaccines at its factories in the U.S. and Belgium. For the foreseeable future, it would be up to Andreas and his protégés to keep one of the largest clinical trials in medical history supplied with safe and stable vaccines.

For a moment, it had seemed like BioNTech would get a helping hand. In early April, Bill Gates had urged governments to build manufacturing sites in advance of knowing which COVID-19 vaccines, if any, would work. His charitable foundation, he said, would itself invest in plants for seven different candidates. "It'll be a few billion dollars we'll waste on manufacturing for the constructs that don't get picked because something else is better," the Microsoft founder told *Daily Show* host Trevor Noah. "But a few billion in this, the situation we're in, where there's trillions of dollars . . . being lost economically," he added, "is worth it."[1]

Despite the obvious economic and epidemiological imperative, no such scheme materialized. There was no coordinated international effort to identify idle production capacity or build new facilities in preparation for the first authorized vaccines. A playbook for responding to viral outbreaks as a "global coalition" had been developed at the World Economic Forum in Davos in 2000 and was updated in 2017. It fell apart almost as soon as it was exposed to geopolitical reality. Andreas and his staff were on their own.

Most biotechnology companies of BioNTech's size would not have had any manufacturing capacity of their own to begin with. In fact, Uğur and Özlem's first business, Ganymed, had enlisted external contractors to make its monoclonal antibody therapies. Even though working with these companies had proved to be a trying process, when the couple founded BioNTech, they halfheartedly charged Andreas with identifying similar vendors to help the cash-strapped start-up produce mRNA medicines. BioNTech ran so-called feasibility studies with a small American firm, but as neither it nor any contract manufacturer in the world had produced mRNA drugs, Andreas quickly realized that teaching another team about the technology was more trouble than it was worth. Besides, for the process to run smoothly, too much know-how would have to be handed over to a supplier, and some of it could wind up in the hands of competitors. Instead, BioNTech would find a way to make its experimental vaccines and therapies in-house, following the example of fellow German mRNA company CureVac. In late 2008, Andreas traveled to the university town of Heidelberg for a crash course in Good Manufacturing Practice, or GMP, the globally recognized regulations for ensuring consistent quality in the production of licensed pharmaceuticals. At around the same time, Moderna started to develop its own plant in Massachusetts. The nascent mRNA industry was accumulating manufacturing expertise.

Building such facilities from scratch, however, was beyond a young BioNTech's capabilities. Constructing clean rooms and obtaining the necessary approvals to produce clinical material would be a laborious process, one that could take up to three years. Luckily, within months of the company's founding, a GMP-certified site just fifty-five miles to the west of Mainz, which had been losing €2 million a year, came on the market. Uğur and Özlem saw an opportunity to conscript an expert production team and a ready-to-go factory in one fell swoop. Although it would be a while before they needed to manufacture large quantities of mRNA for human trials, the couple—with the blessing of their lead investors, the Strüngmann twins—decided to buy the plant in Idar-Oberstein, which was being offered to them for €2.5 million, and put the thirty-odd employees there on the payroll. The team, which soon became familiar with the peculiarities of mRNA production, expanded significantly over the years. By 2018, the company, needing more capacity than Idar-Oberstein could offer, built a supplementary facility in Mainz and staffed that one too.

It was to those employees that Andreas had turned in early February, once Uğur had told him that "if this is going to get as bad as I think it is, we have to dedicate our entire manufacturing capabilities to COVID-19." Without knowing what dose would be required to prompt an immune response or how many other vaccines would be on the market, Uğur estimated that the company would need to produce a total of 1 kilogram of mRNA—enough for between five to twenty million vaccines, dependent on the final dosage—by the end of 2020. At that point, the most BioNTech had ever manufactured in a year was a tenth of that: 100 grams, usually in 1-gram batches. The maximum material produced in one run was just 8 grams.

Thanks to the vision that Uğur and Özlem had shared as young doctors, decades earlier, BioNTech was ready for such a ramp-up. In the mid-1990s, they learned that all cancers were "highly diverse" and could seldom be targeted by a therapy encoding for a common antigen, or target. "Back then, we understood," Uğur says, "that to enable individualized drugs, we needed a technology that lends itself to versatile manufacturing processes." In effect, what the couple were proposing was to turn the medicine industry on its head. Instead of developing pharmaceuticals that could eventually be mass-produced and benefit from the cost savings of large-scale manufacturing, each patient would get their own, custom-made cure. mRNA, it turned out, was ideally suited for this purpose.

As a result, production at the facilities that Andreas had helped BioNTech acquire needed to be "very fast, very agile, and very adaptable," says Özlem. The tens of thousands of steps involved in mRNA drug-making would have to be repeated for each individualized therapy, and there was no room for error. Patients enrolled in the company's early clinical trials would usually be suffering from late-stage cancer. To work out if the experimental BioNTech drug they had agreed to take was doing the trick, the volunteers would have to stop receiving chemotherapy or other treatments. They did not have the luxury of waiting for months.

Uğur, Özlem, and their teams would rarely meet the beneficiaries of their tailor-made medicines, but occasionally, a patient would reveal themselves to the press, making the acceleration of the process even more personal. Brad Kremer, a fifty-two-year-old sales rep from Massachusetts, was one of those people. He was pictured in *Nature* magazine in a plaid shirt, stroking his pet schnauzer, talking emotionally about "actually witnessing the cancer cells shrinking before [his] eyes," after receiving an experimental, individualized melanoma treatment from BioNTech. It was stories like these that the couple used to motivate manufacturing staff during the early days at Idar-Oberstein. "Each batch," Özlem would say, "is a patient waiting."

The task facing Andreas's team in early 2020 went far beyond the competencies they had developed to cater to such cases. Before the coronavirus emerged in China, BioNTech had planned to sell a maximum of ten thousand doses of its cancer drugs a year, starting in 2024. Now the company would work toward producing millions of doses *per week*. But at least there was a playbook in place, which had been refined and refined. Manufacturing cycles had been reduced from months to weeks, and staff had run through them so many times that they had become adept at problem-solving on the fly. "The batch-release process is the same for individualized and industrial scales," says Oliver Hennig, who makes sure BioNTech's manufacturing facilities run smoothly. "We had the expertise, and we were ready."

BioNTech's bank account, however, was not. Suddenly, everything from enzymes, to nucleotides, to buffers, to bags for bioreactors had to be bought in advance, at enormous cost. Even the 8-gram production runs for cancer products had racked up a six-digit euro bill. Not only would the company now be manufacturing more than eight times that amount in every COVID-19 vaccine batch, but it would have to do several test runs to ensure it could consistently produce the drug to a certain quality, adding to the expense. "We were like: 'Probably, we need that. Maybe we need that. We don't know. Let's buy it anyway,'" says Sierk Poetting, BioNTech's chief financial officer.

Making large amounts of mRNA also meant that a single, human mistake—such as the one that would contaminate fifteen million doses of the Johnson & Johnson vaccine in 2021—could lead to vaccine substance worth millions of euros being poured down the drain.

Uğur was also insistent that the company take the risk of buying materials in sufficient quantities for both clinical trials *and* the initial supply of an authorized vaccine, which still seemed a distant dream. As a matter of priority, BioNTech needed to secure enough lipids with which to wrap naked mRNA, and at the time, there was only one vendor producing the precise formulation needed. Avanti, a family-owned firm just outside of Birmingham, Alabama, asked for a €5 million down payment. A purchase order was signed off by Sierk.

Vials, rubbers, stoppers, and caps—all components required for the bottling of the vaccine—needed to be ordered too. "It was a seller's market," says Oliver, and there was "very little competition" among suppliers. "We were trying to buy the glass that AstraZeneca was trying to buy, and vice versa." Millions of euros needed to be spent on booking so-called fill-and-finish capacity, with contractors who would prepare the vaccines for labeling and shipping. BioNTech's meager cash reserves—which had amounted to €600 million at the start of 2020—were rapidly depleting.

Money had been getting tight before Project Lightspeed got going. In early February, while Uğur and Özlem were assembling a coronavirus vaccine team, BioNTech's chief strategy officer, Ryan Richardson, had traveled to the U.S. to raise money from investors by selling additional shares in the company. Thanks to a quirk of the German legal system, however, he failed to drum up enough interest. "It was really a technicality," he explains. Private investors want to buy new stock from biotech companies at a preferential discount, usually of at least 10 percent. While this is normal practice in America (Moderna raised $500 million in February 2020 at a 20 percent discount[2]) it was illegal for BioNTech, registered in Europe's largest economy, to offer more than 5 percent off the market price. One by one, fund managers declined to come on board. "It was disappointing," says Ryan. Many German biotechs would domicile in the Netherlands to avoid precisely such a situation. BioNTech, which had remained rooted in Mainz, "had no choice" but to abide by local law.

Characteristically, Uğur and Özlem were not panicked. Both were confident that investors would look past pricing obstacles once the coronavirus vaccine trials began producing convincing data. "We are spending a lot of our budget on this program," Uğur told a reporter in early March, "and we do that trusting that we will get the financial support needed for this project."

But with the bill for crucial components increasing by tens of millions of euros each week, chairman Helmut Jeggle was increasingly concerned about the long-term health of the company. It was not just that the coronavirus vaccine could fail. Even if safe and effective, it could end up being just one among many successful shots and, as a niche product, would remain unprofitable. Plus, while the agreement was that Pfizer would be responsible for commercialization in the vast majority of countries, Uğur and Özlem wanted BioNTech to sell the vaccine directly to Germany and Turkey. This would mean building a whole new department and a medical affairs unit to look after marketing, sales, corporate, and governmental affairs as well as recruiting pharmacovigilance specialists to manage the reporting of adverse events.

Realizing that the capital markets were not coming to BioNTech's aid, Helmut began working his network and secured an introduction to Mariya Gabriel, the commissioner responsible for innovation and research in the European Union. He provided a short presentation to her office, in which he underlined the urgency of the company's undertaking and laid out its costs. Gabriel promised to consider his request.

Meanwhile, on March 15, the subject of EU support for German vaccine developers suddenly hit the headlines. A front-page splash in the Sunday newspaper *Welt am Sonntag*[3] claimed that Donald Trump, who just days before had proclaimed that COVID-19 was "going to disappear," had tried to lure mRNA company CureVac after its chief executive took part in a televised roundtable at the White House on March 2. Much to the alarm of Angela Merkel's government, the article said the president had offered up to a billion dollars to the Tübingen-based business to secure its proposed COVID-19 vaccine exclusively for the United States.

Furious politicians lined up to condemn the alleged move. "Germany is not for sale," economy minister Peter Altmaier told the country's main TV channel, even though both CureVac and, curiously, the Trump administration went on record to say the approach had never taken place. Whether accurate or not, the *Welt* report spooked European leaders. By the evening of Monday, March 16, EU commission president Ursula von der Leyen had called CureVac and offered the company—which had already been funded by the Coalition for Epidemic Preparedness Innovations, or CEPI, back in January—up to €80 million in financial support.[4] The cash, she said, was "to scale up development and production of a vaccine against the corona-virus *in Europe*." What was supposed to be a collaborative, cross-border effort to battle a deadly disease had suddenly become overtly political.

BioNTech, which announced blockbuster deals with China's Fosun and Pfizer on consecutive days following the *Welt* report, did not hear di-rectly from Von der Leyen. But that, Uğur says, was hardly the fault of the EU. In the eyes of many global bodies, BioNTech was mainly a cancer company, devoted to individualized therapies and unlikely to be among the first to come up with a mass-market COVID-19 vaccine in the mid-dle of a pandemic. Plus, outsiders would have fairly surmised that with two large partners on board, hundreds of millions of euros had been put on the table to accelerate BioNTech's vaccine development, and further funding was not currently needed.

In any case, the couple, who had always avoided making promises without knowing if they could keep them, wanted to limit outside inter-ference in the Lightspeed project. They had deliberately kept the scheme secret for as long as possible, disclosing it only when market regulations demanded. They were happy to let lawmakers' perceptions stand.

The first example of this reticence came on March 20, when, five days after the story on CureVac was published, Uğur and Sierk were asked to join a call with Angela Merkel's office, the Kanzleramt. By now, the number of COVID-19-related deaths worldwide was nearing fifteen thousand, and the European Union accounted for almost a third of the morbid total.[5] The German government had instructed the country's army, the Bundeswehr, to build an emergency hospital and was scrambling to secure ventilators. The development of a successful vaccine was more vital than ever, and the chancellery was trying to assess how domestic developers were progress-ing. On a videoconference call, Merkel's economic advisor, Lars-Hendrik Röller, politely inquired as to how BioNTech was doing and asked whether Berlin could be of any help.

Uğur "talked him through the situation," Sierk remembers. But instead of reading out a list of demands, he simply said that for now, there was "nothing specific" the Lightspeed team needed. Uğur's only request was one relayed on behalf of his wife. Merkel's administration was discussing the imposition of curfews, and the prospect had alarmed Özlem, whose daily runs were crucial to her well-being. "I will not survive if they ask me not to jog," she had said to Uğur, half in jest, when she heard of the scheduled meeting. "Mr. Röller," Uğur pleaded on the call later, "no matter what lockdown restrictions you implement, *please*, let people go jogging."

Uğur's wish list had not expanded by much a few weeks later, when Jens Spahn, Germany's health minister, called to inquire when BioNTech would be able to bring a vaccine to market. After thanking the center-right politician for taking an interest, Uğur says, "I told him we had a number of vaccine candidates and were preparing to enter a Phase 1 study by the end of April. We could get some preliminary data in June, I said, and that would tell us if we were on the right track." Spahn then asked if BioNTech needed support. "I said, 'Not now,'" Uğur recalls. All the company wanted, he added, was to be left to carry on with its work.

Sierk, however, was still keen to mitigate the financial fallout. He wrote up a four-page pitch, an extension of the one Helmut had given the EU commissioner, outlining what BioNTech would need to get a vaccine to the world by October. He sent it to several governments and to Spahn. "We didn't ask for a billion, and we didn't need a billion," says Sierk. All he requested was €90 million to support the ramp-up of manufacturing, €50 million for production costs, and €140 million to help run clinical studies. But even once BioNTech had launched the first EU trial for a COVID-19 vaccine in April, there were no offers of monetary assistance on the horizon.

In any case, the figures Sierk had provided quickly became underestimates. While he and Helmut, true to their roles, fretted about failure, Uğur and Özlem had been planning for success. If the vaccine received emergency authorization, each batch of mRNA would be a precious, lifesaving commodity. BioNTech needed to do what it could to supplement production at Pfizer's enormous facilities in Puurs, Belgium, and Kalamazoo, Michigan. Its ambitions for 2020 went up to 5 kilograms of mRNA, far more than Idar-Oberstein or Mainz were capable of, combined.

"It was very, very clear in the early summer that we needed more capacity, and *lots* of it," says Oliver Hennig. Among the many challenges of making such large amounts of mRNA was the fact that pure, pressurized ethanol—so flammable that technicians would have to wear special, static-free boots—needed to be used to wrap the active ingredient in lipids. Neither of BioNTech's existing facilities could "handle thousands of liters of buffers or hundreds of liters of ethanol," says Oliver. "You need explosion-safe environments, which we didn't have." The only option was to go back to Uğur and Özlem's original strategy at the dawn of the company's commercial ambitions: find and acquire more production capacity.

A potential solution lay just sixty miles to the northeast of Mainz, in a former medieval settlement called Marburg.

Home to an imposing eleventh-century castle and the world's oldest Protestant university, the small town had played a larger role in the history of immunology than its size or location suggested. In the late 1800s, German vaccine pioneer Emil von Behring moved to Marburg and set up industrial facilities to produce his "antitoxin," the first pharmaceutical to prevent tetanus.

The manufacturing site built for this purpose, named Behringwerke, soon intertwined with the fortunes of the town. In the 1920s and '30s, locals opposed plans for a Mercedes plant, and after the Second World War, the council voted against allowing other companies to base themselves in Marburg, worried that commercial eyesores would ruin its picturesque charm. While nearby Stadtallendorf got Germany's Nutella factory, Marburg prospered solely due to its pharmaceutical pedigree, becoming a global hub for polio vaccine production. Then, in the 1960s, disaster struck.

A handful of researchers at the plant carrying Behring's name, who had been exposed to the tissue of African green monkeys, suddenly developed hemorrhagic fever. Outbreaks occurred simultaneously in laboratories in nearby Frankfurt and in Belgrade, Yugoslavia. Seven died,[6] and the new pathogen—similar in its effects to Ebola—was calculated to be fatal to almost nine out of every ten people infected.[7] Almost immediately, the disease was given a name: the Marburg virus.

The small town, now synonymous with a biological disaster, worked hard to rehabilitate its image. In 2007, it became the home of the first production facility for a cell-based flu vaccine, a new method that avoided fiddling with chicken eggs.[8] Giants such as Novartis and GlaxoSmith-Kline invested in the site, despite its relative remoteness. But when the two companies swapped assets in 2015, with the Swiss group selling its vaccine unit to GSK, while buying the British company's oncology division, Novartis's campus in Marburg gradually became redundant. It was used to produce cell and gene therapies, but this could be done more efficiently at other sites. Some of the on-site staff, seeing the writing on the wall, looked for jobs elsewhere. A few ended up at BioNTech.

In early May, soon after it became abundantly clear that the Mainz manufacturing facilities would be insufficient to fulfill BioNTech's vaccine ambitions, one of those exiles had relayed a rumor to Sierk. Novartis, the informant had heard, wanted to sell its Marburg base and was on the lookout for a buyer. Sierk could hardly believe his luck and immediately told the rest of the board. Sean Marett, in charge of business relationships, sprang into action and approached the Swiss company, only to be rebuffed by management. "The Novartis people were like: 'What the hell are these people on?'" says Sean. "What is an early-stage biotech going to do with a factory if their coronavirus project fails?" Putting hundreds of employees' futures in the hands of a precarious start-up was not a good look for a Big Pharma group, especially if those workers ended up losing their jobs. Concerned about such an eventuality, Novartis brushed Sean off.

The British executive, however, was persistent. Sean secured a meeting with Novartis boss Vas Narasimhan and presented BioNTech's plans to him virtually. But the follow-up emails involved the same middle managers who had rejected the company's approach in the first place. The offer was once again rebuffed.

While the search for manufacturing sites continued, Sierk and Helmut's fundraising efforts started to pay off. EU commissioner Gabriel organized a €100 million loan from the European Investment Bank, announced on June 11. The focus, however, soon shifted to CureVac. On June 15, German economics minister Peter Altmaier called a press conference in Berlin and revealed that his government was investing €300 million to acquire almost a quarter of the business. In direct reference to the reported approach from the Trump administration, Altmaier told reporters that the country "does not sell its silverware." Hours later, a letter from the German finance ministry was leaked to the press, in which it was revealed that CureVac was planning to go public in New York in a matter of weeks. The money, it said, was "intended to ensure that the company is not taken over by a foreign investor and that it does not leave the country."

This was the type of interference BioNTech had sought to avoid, but it would soon find itself caught in political cross fire too. On June 18, as the dust settled following the news of state intervention in CureVac, Sierk traveled to Berlin to meet German health minister Jens Spahn's team. "It was the first time I took a train again," says the executive, who had been stuck at home in Munich with his kids since early March. "It was scary—I was wearing a mask and squeezing into a corner of the carriage." Upon his arrival at the ministry, Sierk was ushered to a room in which two senior civil servants were sat socially distanced around a light oak table, alongside Sierk's fellow board member Sean and comms chief Jasmina Alatovic.

By this point, the German government, tired of waiting for the EU to make a move, had begun to buy up vaccine supply on its own. Alongside Italy, France, and the Netherlands, it had just signed a deal with Oxford/AstraZeneca for up to four hundred million doses and was considering adding BioNTech to the mix. After some chitchat about the state of the company's clinical trials, the conversation turned to money. AstraZeneca was charging around two euros a dose, the civil servants said. How much, they wanted to know, would their homegrown vaccine cost?

This was a question BioNTech itself was struggling to answer. Before Pfizer had even come on board, Uğur and Özlem had told their teams to pursue a "fair pricing" framework. Those that could afford to pay, such as the U.S. and EU, were to be charged the most, while middle-income countries were to pay roughly half. Fees from wealthier nations would help subsidize supply of the vaccine for developing nations, who would be able to purchase doses almost at cost.

To avoid being deemed a cartel under competition law, BioNTech and Pfizer—separate companies, after all—were not allowed to agree on specific prices in their respective markets. There could be no legal mechanism by which one was able to stop the other charging what it liked. But a principle could be defined, and Uğur's was simple. As he communicated in his first call with Albert Bourla: price shouldn't be a barrier to global vaccine supply.

Matters became more complicated at the end of April after AstraZeneca signed a deal to help develop the Oxford vaccine. The Anglo-Swedish group's chief executive, Pascal Soriot, told the *Financial Times* newspaper[9] that the company—which had posted an operating profit of almost $6 billion in 2019—was committed to providing the product at cost during the pandemic, piling pressure on Pfizer to do the same. But while the giant U.S. pharmaceutical company could easily follow suit, BioNTech, which would swallow half of the costs of Project Lightspeed, could not.

In the years preceding the company's flotation on the Nasdaq, its losses had ballooned. At the end of 2018 BioNTech had accumulated a deficit of more than €245 million. Twelve months later, that number had grown to €425 million. This was by no means unusual for a venture-capital-financed biotech, which needed to survive for long enough to reach the final stages of drug development. But by the time it started working on a COVID-19 vaccine, the company was sitting on almost half a billion euros of debt.[10] Faced with the prospect of birthing the first-ever commercial mRNA product, BioNTech could ill afford to undersell its invention.

The idea of providing the vaccine at cost to industrialized countries was not entertained. It was important to Uğur and Özlem for the money made from a coronavirus vaccine—built on a technology that had been developed for cancer treatments—to flow back into the company's oncology pipeline. "COVID is an emergency," Uğur had told commercialization manager Michael Böhler, "but cancer is the bigger killer." Chairman Helmut Jeggle was of a similar mind. "There must be a reward for innovation," he says, recalling his stance in those months, "otherwise, you end up with average." The issue was, at least internally, settled. BioNTech would not engage in profiteering, but it would not apologize for seeking to make a profit.

When Sierk and Sean were called to meet the German government in Berlin in June, however, they knew civil servants would want more than principles—they would want an indicative price. A day before their trip, the board had held an impromptu virtual meeting to discuss what they would communicate. "We did not know what the cost of raw materials would be, we did not know the size of dose, and we did not know how many doses we could get from each production batch," says Uğur, "so I preferred to say nothing about the price. But the EU [via Germany] was pressuring."

Reluctantly, the board came up with a negotiating position, one that covered their highest evaluation of the expenses involved in producing the vaccine. "We went in with €54 something per dose," says Sierk, believing that estimate would come down significantly when a winning candidate and dose was chosen, manufacturing processes put in place, and ingredients ordered in bulk. The ballpark figure would come back to haunt BioNTech, when the *Süddeutsche Zeitung* newspaper revealed it to the public in February 2021,[11] and jeering commentators pointed to the unfortunate address of the company's headquarters: An der Goldgrube, or "at the gold mine" (which was actually a reference to a Roman find). But if the civil servants in the sweltering health ministry on that June afternoon were shocked by the estimate, they did not let it show. "They just said they would take it back to their superiors," Sierk remembers. Half an hour later, he boarded a half-empty Deutsche Bahn train and returned to Munich.

The mood music changed less than two weeks later, when BioNTech and Pfizer announced to the world, on July 1, that one of their vaccine candidates was triggering a powerful immune response in Phase 1 trial participants. By this point, the companies had analyzed blood samples taken from forty-five volunteers, two dozen of which had received a second shot. Participants double-dosed with 10 micrograms of the modRNA construct expressing the receptor-binding domain part of the spike protein—the same construct that had been tested in-house by Alex Muik at the end of May—were found to have almost twice the level of neutralizing antibodies as recovered COVID-19 patients. Those double-dosed with 30 micrograms had almost *three times as much.*

Now—having an approximate idea of the final vaccine's dose size—the companies could answer the burning question of approximately how many courses they would be able to produce and deliver. Assuming a 30-microgram dose, they said, 100 million shots could be manufactured in 2020, followed by 1.2 billion doses in 2021—enough to fully vaccinate the adult populations of Europe and the U.S. BioNTech's shares jumped by a fifth, and the company's comms team was bombarded with requests from the global press, eager to talk to Uğur and Özlem, and learn more about mRNA.

With production costs also becoming clearer, the pricing of the vaccine could now be privately communicated to interested countries. It would be around €17.50 per shot for those most able to pay, BioNTech told government officials, and slightly more than that for those placing smaller orders.

Britain was the first to sign on the dotted line. Kate Bingham, the venture capitalist appointed by Prime Minister Boris Johnson as the head of the UK's "vaccine task force," was an old friend of Sean's. The two had worked together when she invested in a start-up he had worked at years before joining BioNTech. Immediately after assuming her role in early May, Kate sent Sean a text and, after an initial chat on May 12, followed up with several calls, in which she tried to persuade him to agree to a deal. "I basically hounded him," says the life sciences specialist. With four different mRNA candidates still in clinic, Sean was "not keen on signing any deals until it was clear what he would actually be selling," she says, but on July 20, after it became clear that there was at least one vaccine in Phase 1 trials able to prompt an immune response, a contract for thirty million doses was inked. Project Lightspeed had its first customer.

Over in the U.S., Pfizer received similarly eager inquiries from Operation Warp Speed, the vaccines and therapies task force created by the Trump White House on May 15. It had chosen to back three vaccine technologies and use its $10 billion fund to support two companies in each field. The American government was already working with Moderna, and Moncef Slaoui, the veteran pharmaceuticals executive appointed to run Warp Speed, wanted to invest directly in Pfizer's vaccine project too, essentially co-opting the company into the country's coronavirus response. "It was compellingly obvious," Moncef says, "that Moderna and BioNTech were the ones to back."

Albert Bourla, however, was adamantly against that form of funding. "It was the Trump administration, with elections [coming up], so the political environment was very, very intense," he recalls. "I knew if we took the money, they [would] want a seat at the table," says the Pfizer boss, who made this decision without talking to Uğur. He had not wanted to "burden [his] scientists with this bureaucracy."[12] Instead, Albert told Moncef he wanted to negotiate a straightforward purchase agreement with the U.S. Just buy the doses, was the message, and we will supply.

Moncef, who was in close contact with Kate Bingham (and says he hardly ever spoke to any of his EU counterparts), came through two days after the UK, placing an initial order of one hundred million doses, with the option to purchase an additional five hundred million—more than enough to vaccinate the entire adult American population. Both countries acted quickly because their task forces were led by "industry people," says Sean, and both insisted on complete independence from their political masters.

The EU's vaccine procurement team had no such luxury. It was directly accountable to elected officials from twenty-seven member states, some of whom favored homegrown developers, like France's Sanofi and Valneva. Negotiators, knowing that much of their work could be made public if parliamentarians requested their correspondence, were hesitant to back an unproven mRNA vaccine, for which real-world efficacy data was still lacking, and did not place an early order. "There was no blueprint for procurement in a pandemic," says Özlem, reflecting on the approach a year later, "so it was not a surprise that the EU needed some time to survey the landscape."

The bloc's resources were also much smaller. Despite the EU having a larger population than the U.S., Europe's vaccine task force (alongside a fund that previously tackled forest fires and other natural disasters[13]) was endowed with roughly $3.2 billion,[14] just under a third of the funds available to Warp Speed. Less wealthy EU countries were demanding to know why Brussels would entertain using this meager budget for a relatively expensive vaccine, when cheaper ones using more established methods would likely be available. Others were frustrated by the constant nickeling-and-diming, notably Germany. It was part of the quartet of member states—including France, Italy, and the Netherlands—that had started to unilaterally procure vaccines, only to be reined in by President Ursula von der Leyen. But after the U.S. and UK signed supply deals, this group wanted the EU task force to follow suit—fast. "Sometimes it seemed to me the commission was representing twenty-seven different views," says Sean, who dealt directly with the EU's negotiators. As a result, even as BioNTech's vaccine looked poised to be the first in Europe to enter the final phase of clinical studies, no doses had been bought by the EU. "I try not to be too critical," Sean says of the drawn-out procurement process, "but we were on our own."

Uğur, who seldom criticizes people or institutions, had a more nuanced view. "I sensed what was going on behind the scenes," he says. "But I knew it would soon be clear that our vaccine was worth ordering. I asked Sean to keep the door open for the EU."

Months later, the EU officials' nervousness about making bold bets would, ironically, seem justified by a series of public outcries over clauses in contracts it signed with vaccine manufacturers, perhaps sensing that there was a prolonged dispute over who would be responsible in the unlikely event that the vaccine ended up harming healthy people. A slew of lawsuits could dent the figures of a giant pharma company, but for a biotech, they could prove fatal. To oil the wheels in a public health emergency, Britain and the U.S. had waived limits on manufacturers' liability, while the EU had agreed to indemnify AstraZeneca for such an eventuality. But the bloc was scornful of sharing risk with BioNTech and Pfizer. "Their benchmark was: AstraZeneca is only charging us x, and you want significantly more per dose, so you should take more liability," says Sean. The company, he responded, "can't afford to sell to you at that price, and if we sell at the AstraZeneca price, we won't be able to do this at the next pandemic, because we won't exist."

In 2021, after hundreds of millions of people had been vaccinated, researchers in the U.S. and UK would attempt to calculate what each dose was worth to the world economy. Their results would put the haggling over euros and cents into unflattering perspective. Three billion "annual vaccine courses," the academics would write, have "a global benefit of $17.4 trillion." Per inoculated person, they would estimate, the average benefit was a whopping $5,800.[15]

The political heat of vaccine procurement was matched only by the soaring temperatures within the Şahin and Türeci household. The family's small apartment featured many glass windows, and with Mainz experiencing July highs of 35 degrees Celsius, it soon felt like a greenhouse. "We expected Frodo to come to the door and throw a ring in," says Özlem, referring to the volcano of Mount Doom in the *Lord of the Rings* saga.

The news coming through from the couple's colleagues, however, had a cooling effect. As Uğur had expected, the encouraging Phase 1 data had captured the attention of the financial markets. On the second time of asking, Ryan Richardson managed to execute a capital raise, using an innovative deal structure to avoid a repeat of February's failure. By the end of the month, BioNTech had fetched more than half a billion dollars from new and existing investors, plus a further quarter of a billion from a fund run by the government of Singapore.

BioNTech and Pfizer also sealed further supply deals with Japan, Canada, and several smaller states. Israel paid a premium to be ahead of the queue when it came to delivery and offered to share anonymized health data from its population of nine million. There would be no shortage of takers for the companies' vaccine, if, of course, it proved to be effective.

One of BioNTech's vaccine candidates looked likely to fulfill that mission. The B.1, whose data had been announced on July 1, had survived what Pfizer's Kathrin Jansen coined the "quick kill" strategy, in which the uRNA and saRNA constructs tested in the Phase 1 study had been eliminated. Although it caused a fever in three-quarters of those who were given it, it was the construct that led the UK, the U.S., and several others to order doses up front, and the one that had convinced investors to put money on the table. It was also to be used in an upcoming Phase 1 study in China, run by Fosun, which had taken weeks and weeks to get into shape.

There was, however, a straggler. Like B.1, it was built on the modRNA platform, but instead of expressing the small receptor-binding domain of the coronavirus, it coded for the full spike protein. This was the construct that Uğur had switched out for a newer version, the B2.9, at the very last minute, rearranging production in Idar-Oberstein after Alex Muik's tests showed it prompted better responses in mice. Due to the complexities of the manufacturing process, it had been administered in the first-in-human study a full three weeks after the B.1. The blood samples from patients injected twice with B2.9 would take a while to come through.

With the start of a Phase 3 study scheduled for the end of July, "we quickly came to think that as soon as we get something that flies, we are probably going to go ahead with it, because of the imperative of the pandemic, even if it means we don't find the best candidate," says Martin Bexon, a consultant who helped run the German first-in-human study. After all, Claudia Lindemann had pulled out all the stops to reduce the duration of the toxicology study, from six months to two, and Özlem and her team had shaved weeks off the Phase 1 trial's length. A strong vaccine had emerged from these accelerated processes, and supply-chain specialists had come up with a plan to produce tens of thousands of doses for a global clinical trial. With all that had been achieved at "Lightspeed," could BioNTech, in possession of a candidate that flew, afford to sit on its hands and wait?

For Uğur and Özlem, the answer was a resounding *yes*. First, data had been trickling in from BioNTech's studies, and those carried out by other vaccine developers, showing that vaccines encoding for the full spike, like B2.9, were not causing antibody-dependent enhancement—ADE— the potentially dangerous phenomenon that had kept the couple up at night when they first embarked on Project Lightspeed. One of the reasons they had included B.1, which targeted the smaller receptor-binding domain, in the Phase 1 finalists was to mitigate the chances of this dreaded effect, which had plagued early efforts to create vaccines against SARS and MERS, and which, as we learned in chapter 3, had harmed American children injected with an RSV inoculation in the 1960s. Now that it was becoming clear that ADE was not an issue in a SARS-CoV-2 vaccine, a construct that expressed the full spike—like the B2.9—was more attractive. It would give the forces of the immune system a larger area to target and might be better at disrupting the powerful docking mechanism the virus uses to infiltrate cells.

The B2.9 would also, the doctors suspected, be able to summon T-cells—those specialist sharpshooters of the immune army that apply the "kiss of death" to diseased cells—in greater numbers. There were good reasons to believe that these snipers, which Uğur and Özlem had spent decades directing toward cancers, would be crucial to combating the coronavirus too. By the end of March, publications had shown that some people who got COVID-19 but only suffered mild symptoms had T-cell responses but no antibodies, pointing to the increased importance of this second line of defense.

Large pharmaceutical companies, however, "did not appreciate how important T-cell data [is]," says Özlem. For some pathogens, antibodies, which attack *before* a virus manages to enter cells, are enough to prevent infection, but not for all, and certainly not for coronaviruses. Yet antibodies took precedence for most developers. "The infectious disease vaccine industry has developed this way; I don't understand it," Özlem adds. Convincing Pfizer to hang on for T-cell data would not be easy.

Uğur had foreseen such an eventuality. "We had a very clear understanding with Kathrin," he says, "that we are not going to jump on the first vaccine that works." She agreed to wait.

As the teams on either side of the Atlantic waited for more data on the B2.9, supply-chain managers, concerned that there would now not be sufficient vaccine to meet the demands of the Phase 3 study, grew increasingly irate. Tens of thousands of participants needed to be dosed at dozens of centers worldwide, and manufacturing that much material with several weeks' head start was hard enough. Changing the candidate just days before launch, they warned, was a bridge too far.

Uğur soon found a way of placating them. It was based, once again, on math. He had noticed a disparity between the amount of vaccine being produced for the Phase 1 studies in the U.S. and Germany, and the amounts actually administered to volunteers. Although sufficient quantities were being delivered, the clinicians were often short of supply. What Uğur realized was that due to strict handling instructions, up to 80 percent of the 0.5 milliliters of vaccine in each vial was being wasted. Since the drug did not contain preservatives, doctors and nurses were only allowed to use it for six hours after a vial had been opened, to avoid contamination from bacteria. They were getting two or three doses out of the small bottles, but as trial participants were coming in for their injections at different points in the day, often separated by more than six hours, the rest was thrown away.

Uğur emailed his finding to the BioNTech and Pfizer teams, along with a suggestion. Each vial should contain *less* vaccine, he said, with the filling volume reduced to 0.3 milliliters. The manufacturing would be a little more complicated, but with 60 percent more vials being produced, fewer doses would ultimately go to waste, he argued. With just two weeks to go until the Phase 3 was due to start, Pfizer's operations teams countered that it was too late to change such details. Uğur then called Kathrin Jansen, and said, "I really need you to support this," only to be told that the U.S. giant had standard procedures in place that were difficult to alter at the last minute. "With changes in process comes risk," Kathrin remembers saying. Eventually, however, Pfizer saw the advantages too, and after several phone calls, the alteration was agreed.

Data on the B2.9 soon began trickling in. When it came to neutralizing antibodies, Alex Muik's tests showed that the vaccine was almost as good as its modRNA sibling, the B1. It also seemed to be better tolerated by trial participants, with side effects like fever being observed less frequently. Then, on July 23, less than twenty-four hours before Decision Day, the much-awaited T-cell data came through. An image had been produced not too dissimilar to the one full of purple dots that Uğur and Özlem's team had seen on a screen on the fateful day in 2004, which proved that certain dendritic cells in lymph nodes were particularly adept at hoovering up mRNA. It showed that, as suspected, the candidate was bringing both types of T-cells to the fight and bringing them out in greater force than the B1 had. It proved B2.9, the modRNA encoding for the full spike, was "an almost perfect vaccine, from an immunological standpoint," Uğur told a friend shortly afterward, marshaling all the immune system's army units simultaneously, and raising his hopes that, together, they would defeat SARS-CoV-2. "It is easy to say we will be guided by science and data, but you need the strength to stick to that," said an unusually emotional Uğur, who was convinced that the decision to wait for B2.9 would, in a few months' time, change the course of the pandemic. He repeated what he had told his newly assembled coronavirus vaccine team when he had given them their initial instructions in early February: "Science is first, speed a close second."

Not everyone shared Uğur and Özlem's zeal for B2.9. First, there was still some missing data on how the construct worked on older people—the group most vulnerable to COVID-19. This cohort had been dosed last in the Phase 1 trials, at the regulators' insistence, and it was too early to take the blood tests from the over-fifty-fives injected with B2.9. Second, while Pfizer's head of vaccines, Kathrin Jansen, and her deputy, Phil Dormitzer, were convinced by the supremacy of this candidate, others at the U.S. giant, not all that used to caring about T-cell responses, felt that antibodies were the more important measure, and B1 prompted these troops to deploy in marginally greater force.

BioNTech did not *need* to reach a consensus on this issue. One of the few rights that it had preserved after that videoconference in which Uğur had given away most decision-making powers—causing business-development ace Roshni to swear silently to herself—was the final say on candidate selection for the Phase 3 study. But Uğur did not want to force anything through, and so an enormous Zoom call was scheduled for July 24, three days before the final-stage trial was due to kick off. Sixty people were invited. All knew the virtual meeting had to end in a resolution.

Uğur and Özlem joined from home, as did BioNTech's regulatory expert Ruben Rizzi, manufacturing lead Andreas Kuhn, and test supremo Alex Muik, among others. A "cast of thousands" from Pfizer dialed in too, including the clinical leads for the Phase 3 study, Bill Gruber and Steve Lockhart, and regulatory head Donna Boyce. Among the senior representatives from the pharma group were Kathrin and Phil and chief scientific officer Mikael Dolsten. "We knew that we would put a billion dollars at risk now, with no return," Mikael recalls. In his own words, the Swedish-born scientist says he tried to take a step back and say: "Look, the thing that is in front of us we know less, but it has more data pointing in the right direction."[16]

After an hour of to-and-fro, the group came to an agreement.

BioNTech and Pfizer would put their combined efforts, and fortunes, on B2.9—or to give it its full code name: BNT162b2.9.

Out of the twenty candidates that had entered Project Lightspeed's labyrinth in February, four had been clinically tested. At the end of May, one had shown promise. Now, just six months after Uğur sat at his desk and read the article about asymptomatic spread in *The Lancet*, an "almost perfect" candidate had emerged. "The Vaccine" was born.

A billion-dollar question, however, remained unanswered. Would the virus develop a mechanism to escape the immune system's grasp? The B2.9, Uğur told colleagues at the time, was "as good as it gets" when it came to calling on specialist forces: antibodies and T-cells. But there was still a chance that SARS-CoV-2 would win the evolutionary arms race. "We don't know the other side of the equation," Uğur said. "We don't know how the enemy will behave."

To find out, the companies launched their large-scale Phase 3 trial on July 27, intending to enroll thirty thousand volunteers in Germany, and the U.S. Pfizer's experienced clinical operations team oversaw the logistics of the study itself, recruiting participants, making sure each was given two shots, three weeks apart, and monitoring for side effects. Andreas Kuhn's team worked in back-to-back shifts in Idar-Oberstein and Mainz, once again manufacturing just enough mRNA to keep the show on the road.

Soon, however, their heroic efforts would be insufficient. To answer the billion-dollar question of whether the vaccine worked in the real world, a significant portion of study volunteers would have to be exposed to infection. But thanks to lockdowns, mask wearing, and other public health measures, the virus was being somewhat suppressed in America and Europe. The study had to be expanded to countries where the pandemic was still raging, and sites in Brazil, Argentina, South Africa, and Turkey were added, stretching the total number of recruits to well over forty thousand.

"As they opened up more and more clinical sites, it was not unusual that we received a call from Uğur, asking if we could up the manufacturing," says Andreas. This was much easier said than done. Each batch of vaccine made for clinical trials took between four and six weeks to be ready for injection in humans. First, DNA templates needed to be produced in a lab, an intricate and inconsistent process. Then Andreas's team would translate the DNA into mRNA using bioreactors the size of a student-party beer keg, before purifying the material using buffers, bagging it, and freezing the drug substance at minus 70 degrees Celsius. The plastic sacks—containing enough liquid for a couple of thousand doses—would be placed in specialized Styrofoam boxes roughly as big as a suitcase, but containing dry ice, and handed to a dedicated driver. He would then embark on an eight-hour journey to Polymun in Austria—often overnight—armed with official documents in case he was stopped at the partially closed border, before driving back to do it all again as soon as the next batch was ready.

Once the drug substance arrived at the family-run contractor, it would be thawed before being wrapped in lipids, poured into vials, and capped. This process took a further couple of days, but the most convoluted stage was still to come. A specialist company was needed to properly label the vials, pack them into boxes, and attach a digital thermometer, which would constantly record the temperature, to ensure it did not rise significantly during transit. BioNTech, which had thought at the start of 2020 that it was years away from making its first marketable product, had only vetted one vendor capable of completing all these tasks. The company was Almac, and it was based in County Armagh, Northern Ireland.

Since there was no time to audit another facility, the vials filled at Polymun in Vienna had to be frozen, put in dry ice boxes again, and placed on the back of a truck to begin a two-day journey across Germany, France, the English Channel, England, Wales, the Irish Sea, Ireland, and finally across Northern Ireland, to Craigavon. While this logistical choreography was being carried out, a series of tests were underway on some held-back doses to ensure the batch of vaccine being transported was of a high enough quality and, crucially, that it was sterile. Only once the all clear was given could the vials be flown from Almac to the sites where volunteers were being dosed.

Not every batch was successful. Even with the expertise BioNTech had gained, just one of the fifty thousand stages of drug production needed to go wrong for doses to be deemed unusable. The dud runs were especially personal for Christoph Prinz, who had only joined BioNTech at the start of 2020 and was leading a team that checked each batch of mRNA to ensure it was of a consistent quality. His younger brother, a doctor, was working in the intensive care unit of a Stuttgart hospital, and would report back at the end of each exhausting shift. "I was trying to develop a vaccine and he would call me at midnight and tell me what was happening," says Christoph. "He was starting to intubate patients, seeing them dying." During one of those discussions, Christoph's brother said he had been forced, in the space of a few hours, to tell three families that their loved ones were gone, after experimental treatments like antivirals had failed to work. "I was sitting there thinking," the manager recalls, "am I doing enough? Can we do better here?"

While not as close to the coalface of COVID-19, others were sharing Christoph's burden. Uğur himself started calling around, trying to accelerate the production process. He phoned Polymun's Dietmar Katinger at 9:00 p.m. on a Friday in August, while the chief executive, who was taking a short break, was on a sailing boat off the coast of a small Greek island. "He asked if we could speed up a release and if I could call the head of our quality assurance," says Dietmar, referring to the checks that needed to be done before doses could be delivered to the Phase 3 administration centers.

By the end of August, Pfizer was lending a hand too. Since there were very few passenger planes, which also carry cargo in their bellies, flying back and forth between Europe and the U.S., Albert Bourla's private jet was sent to Frankfurt to help deliver drug substance.

Christoph Prinz and his colleagues were soon provided with some relief, at least when it came to the daunting task of supplying an authorized vaccine to the world. Following July's positive Phase 1 readout, executives at Novartis agreed to come back to the table and discuss a sale of its Marburg site. On September 17, a portion of the hub built by Emil von Behring with the award money from his Nobel Prize became BioNTech's. In the building from which the immunology pioneer ran his operations, with a bust of the great man behind him, Uğur told the press that once up and running, the plant would be able to churn out 750 million doses of vaccine a year. During a global catastrophe, the town that had become synonymous with a deadly virus was to restore its glory as the global provider of a revolutionary, lifesaving drug.

Specialist equipment was immediately moved in, and Mainz's manufacturing experts were sent over to train Novartis's three hundred staff, who were delighted to be a part of what was by now, clearly, one of the front-running COVID-19 vaccine projects. "There is nothing better than being at the helm and being able to do something to make things better," said Valeska Schilling, a long-standing production manager at Marburg,[17] who learned about mRNA production in a matter of weeks. A Polymun employee also traveled to the site a few weeks later to talk the new team through the lipid formulation process that the company had perfected. Safety checks still needed to be performed and licenses from local authorities obtained, but BioNTech was completing a journey that began twelve years earlier, in pursuit of individualized cancer therapies. Andreas's team had gone from manufacturing milligrams of material to kilograms. Industrialized mRNA production was about to become a reality.

Two days before the Marburg announcement, Berlin finally provided some backing to BioNTech in the form of a €375 million grant. By then, the company had spent a couple of hundred million euros of its own money on raw materials and manufacturing, establishing Europe's first dedicated COVID-19 vaccine production site without so much as a pre-order from the EU itself. Aside from an advance purchase of doses, it would have been useful, says Oliver Hennig, if the bloc had said, "Okay, we will buy enough fill-and-finish capacity for our region, and we'll give it to whoever is leading." Instead, companies had been left to compete over limited resources.

Months later, President Von der Leyen herself would admit to the German paper *Süddeutsche Zeitung* that Europe had been too slow to use its powers. "A country on its own can be a speedboat," she would say, but "the EU is more like a tanker."[18] Yet Uğur and Özlem are happy to have stayed out of the way of all such vessels. Being shielded from political demands was a "comfortable situation" for BioNTech, says Uğur, who does not have "any real complaints" about how the company was treated by European lawmakers. The Lightspeed team had managed to design, test, and mass-produce a vaccine in under eight months, while avoiding all external pressures. And that is how the couple had always wanted it.

Over in the U.S., however, Pfizer was encountering the opposite problem: too *much* political interference.

On the morning of Saturday, August 22, Donald Trump, faced with consistently unfavorable polls, fired off a tweet in which he accused the Food and Drug Administration of slowing down the development of coronavirus drugs in an attempt to harm his prospects of winning the looming presidential election. "The deep state, or whoever, over at the FDA is making it very difficult for drug companies to get people in order to test the vaccines and therapeutics," he wrote. "Obviously, they are hoping to delay the answer until after November 3rd." The president, who was also angry at the FDA's decision to withdraw emergency authorization for hydroxychloroquine, an antimalarial that he had touted as a treatment for COVID-19, tagged the organization's commissioner Stephen Hahn in the post, instigating a social media pile-on. Reports soon emerged alleging that the White House was also trying to bypass safety protocols to fast-track the AstraZeneca vaccine.[19] This, the Pfizer team began to realize, was starting to get dangerous.

The situation worsened when Trump, who was on the campaign trail, holding rally after rally to unmasked crowds in packed stadiums, began suggesting that a vaccine could be ready before "a very special date."[20] This was not, strictly speaking, untrue—Albert Bourla had repeatedly said there was a "high likelihood" of filing for approval in October.[21] The date was selected early in Project Lightspeed, when "we didn't have even in our mind the November 3 date of the U.S. election," the Pfizer CEO says, and was chosen to get a vaccine ready before a surge of winter infections. But the suggestion from Trump that drug development processes were being sped up to suit political priorities would, he feared, erode public trust in a vaccine.

He was right to be concerned. A survey carried out for the health news website STAT in August 2020 found that 82 percent of Democrats and 72 percent of Republicans thought vaccine approvals would be driven by politics, rather than by science. BioNTech and Pfizer could find themselves in the position of having done all the hard work—having developed a safe and effective vaccine—only for most of the American population to refuse to take it. It was a scenario that Uğur and Albert regularly discussed and felt increasingly obliged to prevent.

In early September, on a flight from Frankfurt to Vienna, Albert—who had taken to wearing masks emblazoned with SCIENCE WILL WIN—relayed his concerns to Uğur. The unlikely pair—a Greek Jew and a Turkish Muslim—had just met for the first time and were on their way to visit Polymun. "It was great to see Albert in person," says Uğur. "He was completely without airs and graces, and we spent quite a while talking about our lives, family, and children." While the two were in the air, the conversation turned to heavier matters. Albert revealed that he had been working on a rebuke to Trump and said he would appreciate Uğur's support. From his pocket, he pulled out a folded A4 paper, with a draft title: "The COVID-19 Vaccine-Maker Pledge."

Leaning back in his plane seat, Uğur began scanning through the document. "We, the undersigned biopharmaceutical companies," it read, "want to make clear our ongoing commitment to developing and testing potential vaccines for COVID-19 in accordance with high ethical standards and sound scientific principles." The letter went on to guarantee that the signatories would not cut corners on safety, nor seek to circumvent regulatory requirements. It did not mention Trump by name, but the subtext was glaringly obvious. The bosses of Johnson & Johnson, AstraZeneca, GlaxoSmithKline, Merck, Moderna, Novavax, and Sanofi had agreed to sign, Albert said. Would BioNTech join them?

Despite his lifelong reluctance to engage in political debates, Uğur did not hesitate. "I said to him, 'Thank you, Albert, this is great,'" he remembers. A few days later, the pledge was headline news. Within hours of the letter being published, real-world evidence of the fact that science was in control came from the Oxford/AstraZeneca trial, which was temporarily paused due to an adverse reaction in a volunteer in the UK.

With the coronavirus moving quickly around the world, BioNTech and Pfizer expanded their Phase 3 study to forty-three thousand, making it one of the largest human trials ever run. Now, with October looming, the companies were getting closer to the moment of truth.

Most randomized clinical studies are constructed in the same beautifully simple way. Volunteers either receive a placebo or the drug being tested, but neither they nor anyone involved in the trial is told who got what. Only on a secure database, accessible to independent statisticians and a board of external experts, are the barcodes of the vials assigned to particular trial participants. With this double-blind method in place, the study's sponsors, or instigators, sit back and wait.

What they are waiting for depends on decisions taken with the responsible regulator. In BioNTech and Pfizer's case, the FDA had been very clear about what it wanted to see before considering a coronavirus vaccine for emergency authorization. To work out whether the shot reached the agency's threshold of being more than 50 percent effective in preventing severe disease or death, the American authority wanted at least 164 double-dosed participants to have contracted COVID-19. The external experts would review how many of those cases were among those who had been double-jabbed and how many had received a harmless saline solution, and use the split to calculate how effective the vaccine was.

BioNTech, Pfizer, and the FDA had agreed on a series of interim analyses, when 32, 62, 92, and 120 cases had been confirmed. At each point, if the readout was encouraging, the experts would be able to tell the world that it was mission accomplished, and the companies could start the process of submitting the vaccine for authorization, without waiting for the rest of the cases to be detected.

It was the first of these pit stops that Albert Bourla repeatedly told the media had a "good chance" of being reached by the end of October, even though, as with every trial of such a size, the threshold was a bit of a movable feast, dependent on factors like how quickly cases in Brazil or South Africa were verified and communicated to Pfizer's teams. By now, the prediction was being constantly touted by Trump in TV interviews and at campaign events. During his first chaotic debate with Joe Biden, on September 29 in Cleveland, Ohio, the president said a vaccine was "weeks away."

As those weeks passed, however, that date began to slip, leading Albert to pen another open letter in which he sought to clear up the "great deal of confusion" about the steps needed for vaccine approval. The Pfizer boss softened his guidance, saying that "we may know whether or not our vaccine is effective by the end of October"[22] and the company had to "wait for a certain number of cases to occur, this data may come earlier or later based on changes in the infection rates." On October 27, he told analysts, "We don't have the thirty-two events right now," and the end of the month came and went without a readout. With Election Day drawing near, the rumor mill went into overdrive.

Somewhere along the way, says Pfizer's Kathrin Jansen, the FDA began to voice concern about the interim thresholds. "Are you sure you want to do thirty-two?" she remembers the regulator asking, while pointing out that other developers were choosing to start their first analysis once there was a greater number of confirmed infections. Choosing to "unblind" a trial—to allow an external committee to see how many of those who caught COVID-19 had been double-vaccinated and how many had received a placebo—at such a low number could offer an unreliable assessment of efficacy, the FDA warned. "It was for me a public health issue to go to a bigger number of cases," says Albert, who was worried that if the first results showed an "an efficacy of 56 percent," the public would lose confidence in the vaccine, even if subsequent data showed it to be more effective.

Together, Pfizer and the FDA agreed to wait until at least sixty-two cases were confirmed before releasing efficacy data—a change that would almost certainly push the announcement beyond the U.S. presidential election. "Scientifically, it was the *right* decision to make," says Operation Warp Speed's Moncef Slaoui, who believes a smaller cohort may also not have been representative of society as a whole and would contain too few ethnic minorities to win the trust of communities scarred by the history of their ancestors being medically abused and experimented upon in the United States.[23] He insists he does not know if there were any political considerations behind the choice, but "pragmatically, from a vaccine acceptance standpoint, it was a *critical* decision to make."

The delay, of course, did not go down well with the Trump White House. In the days before Americans went to the polls, the president, who had just survived a brush with COVID-19 himself, summoned Moncef to explain the extended timeline. For weeks, he had been telling the commander in chief that trials could only proceed at the speed of science and that the companies would have to wait until a sufficient number of people were confirmed to have contracted the coronavirus before an efficacy rate could be calculated. He had even told Trump that he did not understand why Albert Bourla had, at one stage, issued predictions on when that moment might come. "I can't tell you when [the data will be publicized], and nobody can tell you when," he claims to have told the president. Moncef, who had previously threatened to resign if there was even a hint of interference in the vaccine authorization process, says he also explained the scientific justification for waiting on sixty-two cases. When asked if Pfizer was playing politics by postponing an announcement, he replied, "With all due respect, Mr. President, I don't care."

IT WORKS!

Let what matters most be said
We may win yet and live

—Surendra Munshi's "Ode to Mainz,"[1]
composed upon news of a successful vaccine

It was the Sunday following Donald Trump's loss, and the collective sigh of relief from health workers and scientists was almost audible. Yes, the number of new coronavirus cases in the U.S. had broken records for four days in a row, peaking at almost 130,000 on Saturday, and yes, Anthony Fauci, the country's leading infectious diseases expert, had told the country it was in for "a whole lot of hurt."[2] But in his victory speech, President-Elect Joe Biden had promised to take on the pandemic with a plan "built on a bedrock of science," calming the frayed nerves of those on the front line. Their crucial work would soon be coordinated by a dedicated task force, committed, in Biden's words, to "getting COVID under control."

Over in Germany, however, Uğur and Özlem were anything but calm. Instead, the normally unflappable couple found themselves in a state of unprecedented anxiety.

Their trepidation had little to do with the changing guard at the White House. Sometime in the next few hours, the doctors knew, an independent committee would deliver its first assessment of their vaccine's efficacy. The number of infections needed to perform a proper assessment—which had been upped from thirty-two to sixty-two, much to Trump's chagrin—had almost certainly been surpassed a few days earlier, but it had taken a while for the tests to be double-checked by clinicians from Berlin to Buenos Aires. Now, in their living rooms around the world, a group of experts, who had been meeting on a weekly basis throughout the trial, were "unblinding" the COVID-19 cases among study participants to see how many of those hit by the disease were double-vaccinated and how many had received a placebo. They would soon calculate whether Project Lightspeed had fulfilled its purpose: to create a working vaccine against a virus holding the world hostage.

Thus far, the trickiest part of the project, the study involving tens of thousands of volunteers in six countries, had, remarkably, gone off with hardly a hitch. The trial had recruited volunteers at an unprecedented pace, even as it was forced to follow the virus around the world as waves of infection peaked and troughed. BioNTech had transformed from a company that had produced a few thousand drug doses in almost twelve years to one that manufactured tens of thousands of vaccines in a matter of weeks. Teams of technicians at its Austrian supplier, Polymun, had worked in round-the-clock shifts to wrap the mRNA with lipids and prepare the material for transportation to approximately 150 trial centers around the globe.

Unlike AstraZeneca, Johnson & Johnson, and Eli Lilly, who, following normal procedures, had temporarily paused their late-stage COVID-19 studies to investigate unexplained illnesses among participants,[3] BioNTech and Pfizer had, almost miraculously, witnessed no such events. In fact, volunteers had reported more or less the same mild symptoms as those in the first-in-human study—some pain at the site of injection, headaches, fatigue, and occasionally mild fever—with only 4 percent experiencing side effects severe enough to impede their daily activities. This was almost a perfect experiment, carried out at "Lightspeed." But no one involved—not the scientists, nor the doctors, nor the patients, nor the clinical staff, nor Uğur and Özlem—knew if all the work would prove worthwhile. They had no idea whether the deadly disease caused by this virus could be prevented by a vaccine or whether it would join the plethora of pathogens, such as HIV and malaria, against which humankind had so far failed to adequately protect itself.

Not knowing precisely when this verdict would be delivered, Uğur and Özlem tried to distract themselves with work. "My parents were tense the whole time, and we didn't really talk," their daughter remembers. Her father, who was uncharacteristically struggling to concentrate on anything, started flipping through his favorite motivational quotes, such as "Stop counting the days, but make the days count," an adage he had used to try to discipline himself in the week leading up to this moment of truth. Özlem says she kept herself distracted by doing some long-overdue ironing, which had been somewhat neglected due to the more urgent matters at hand. "My dear, we have done everything humanly possible to build this vaccine," Uğur said, sensing his wife's nervousness. "Now we are at the mercy of biological reality. Whatever we hear later, what counts is that we made an effort."

The call came at around 8:00 p.m. "My mum looked like she was about to burst into tears, and then my dad's phone rang," says the couple's daughter, "and the person on the other end was like, 'Are you alone?'" Pfizer's chief executive, Albert Bourla, was on speakerphone, but Özlem and the teenager nodded eagerly at Uğur, as if to say, *Keep him talking.* "Do you want to know the data?" Albert asked, maintaining the aural equivalent of a poker face. "No," Uğur kidded, his attempt at a joke falling flat. The next few seconds felt like an eternity, until Albert broke the tension, blurting out, "It works!" After pausing for effect, he added, "It works *fantastically.*"

Less than ten months after he and Özlem had—in that very same room—discussed the possibility of developing an mRNA vaccine against an unnamed pathogen in China, their lead candidate had been found to be more than 90 percent effective at preventing disease. A tiny organism that jumped from animal to human had brought the world to a standstill. It had claimed more than one million lives[4] and looked set to claim millions more. A Phase 1 trial had shown that the vaccine was perfectly capable of activating all the forces of the immune system and of doing so profoundly—Uğur had described the immune response as "ideal" in interviews. But the couple had been on tenterhooks, wondering how the enemy, SARS-CoV-2, would behave when ambushed by these troops. Against all odds, scientific endeavor had, they learned, managed to vanquish the virus.

Minutes earlier, Kathrin Jansen, who had retreated to a hotel in the Hudson Valley with her husband for some rest and recuperation, had been sitting in front of her laptop, finishing a late breakfast. Staring out at her from the screen were members of the data and safety monitoring board, a group of external experts, who had dialed in for a videoconference. The panel, who had been analyzing infection data trickling in from BioNTech and Pfizer's enormous Phase 3 trial since October, began diligently going through the methodology they had used to examine results from the blood tests of 94 volunteers—out of 43,538—confirmed to have caught COVID-19, keeping the Pfizer team in unbearable suspense. Then the experts explained the split—only 4 of those infected had been double-dosed with the actual vaccine, the remaining 90 had received a placebo. The math was clear: the vaccine, code-named BNT162b2, had *far* surpassed the FDA's 50 percent threshold for a successful coronavirus inoculation. In fact, it had shot ahead of many common vaccines, including mumps, yellow fever, and rabies, which had all been developed in more relaxed circumstances.

Once the call had ended, Kathrin called Albert, who was sitting in a meeting room at Pfizer's New York headquarters, surrounded by the company's top brass, and delivered the news. "We have a f*****g successful vaccine!" he yelled,[5] punching the air. Champagne was brought in and toasts made. Kathrin, not a woman known for outward displays of emotion, admits to having gotten teary-eyed before enjoying a glass of bubbly too.[6] "Uğur didn't expect, I didn't expect, Kathrin did not expect, no one was expecting that we would be that high," says Albert. "It was the realization that this was a game changer." In Mainz, Uğur and Özlem, who don't drink, brewed some black tea and, after "jumping around the apartment," enjoyed a cake baked by their daughter. "It was a fantastic relief," Uğur remembers. "There was a lot of indication that the vaccine provided immunity," he says "but until that moment, there was no definitive proof."

It was also the first time Uğur and Özlem knew for certain that the vaccine would not cause damage to those who subsequently contracted the disease. The Phase 1 study in Berlin and Mannheim had only demonstrated the safety of the vaccine *itself*, not whether the immune response it provoked would prove too potent in the event of a later infection. In the meantime, tests on primates had shown no indication of ADE, or antibody-dependent enhancement, in which the vaccine helps the virus infect cells. But now there was real-world evidence of its absence. The horror scenarios that had unfolded in Washington in the 1960s, when children who received an RSV vaccine died, and in the animal studies for early SARS and MERS vaccine candidates, which ended up harming the subjects, had not materialized. A cytokine storm, in which overeager foot soldiers in the immune army attacked healthy organs, had also not been observed. There had been six deaths in the Phase 3 study of the coronavirus vaccine, but none were found to be related to the injections. This, Uğur said to Özlem, half in bewilderment, was "a perfect outcome."

Since the end of January, the doctors had woken up each morning with the gnawing thought, never acknowledged out loud, that Project Lightspeed *might* fail miserably, leaving the company they had carefully built mired in debt and putting its cancer pipeline in jeopardy. Now, sitting side by side on their sofa, tea in hand, they talked openly for the first time about the devastation defeat would have wrought. "We had been traveling at the speed of light for months, and now, suddenly, it was as if time stood still," says Uğur. "We allowed ourselves to be emotional and to think about what it would have meant to us, and the team that had worked day and night for months, if we had not been successful." The two scientists also considered the many conscious decisions and chance encounters that had led them to this point. "We thought aloud about what this would mean to the world," says Özlem. "We felt lucky and grateful that nature had proven to be compassionate."

With both Pfizer and BioNTech being publicly listed companies, the couple were barred from sharing the news with anyone other than fellow board members and senior employees before the data was made public. "At that moment, it was the most material information in the world," says Albert, especially as Pfizer planned to submit for emergency authorization with the FDA as soon as possible. Uğur was unable to call Thomas Strüngmann, the couple's benefactor who was about to be handsomely rewarded for his steadfast belief in their abilities. But he did call Helmut Jeggle, BioNTech's chairman, and Michael Motschmann, the investor and supervisory board member who had first introduced Uğur to Thomas. It was 10:00 p.m., and Michael had been pacing the floors, wondering what he would say to Uğur if the results proved disappointing. "I was already thinking, how can I build him up again if things go wrong?" he says. Moments later, his fears were assuaged. "Michael," Uğur said on the phone, "it is even better than we'd thought."

At 12:45 p.m. German time on the following afternoon—Monday, November 9—Pfizer and BioNTech shared the groundbreaking data with the world. The reaction was greater than anyone in either company had expected. Both businesses' shares soared, with billions of dollars added to their market worth. BioNTech became as valuable as the 157-year-old pharmaceuticals giant Bayer, the purveyor of aspirin. Stock markets were lifted too—the S&P 500 opened at a record high in New York, while investors anticipating an end to the pandemic poured money into airlines such as British Airways' parent IAG, and Air France–KLM, causing the price of crude oil to jump sharply.

Personal messages came flooding in to Uğur and Özlem from around the globe. "I get to tell all my friends I know the BioNTech team. We don't generally brag, but we'll brag about this!!!!!!!" read one email from an early investor. "Could be the most important discovery in the last 100 years!!!!" wrote a fellow scientist and decade-long friend, while another texted: "Do celebrate!"

Anthony Fauci, who had hoped for a 75 percent effective vaccine, described the outcome as "just extraordinary" and told reporters the data "validates the mRNA platform." The news, he said, meant it was very likely that other vaccines would also prove efficacious, finally offering humanity a route out of the COVID-19 pandemic. "It validates greatly the spike protein as the target . . . of the immune response," he said, pointing out that most other manufacturers had also chosen to focus on the knobby protrusion. BioNTech and Pfizer may have been "the first out of the gate," but with eleven other vaccines in Phase 3 trials,[7] more would soon follow.

The positive news on the vaccine front also made lockdowns easier to justify for governments, especially in Europe, where a second wave was looming and where, after a summer of relative freedom, restrictions were being reimposed. Germany itself had implemented an "emergency brake" just days earlier, with all restaurants and entertainment venues once again closed, and contacts between households severely limited.[8] But BioNTech's data had given the world a shot of hope; all the public needed was a little more patience.

Mainz, the city that was hitherto most famous for heralding the printing revolution, became the epicenter of a medical one that dominated the front pages worldwide. OUR LITTLE BOTTLE OF HOPE, ran the UK's *Daily Mirror,* accompanied by a picture of the BioNTech vaccine vial. *The Times* headline screamed VACCINE MILESTONE HERALDS "NORMAL LIFE BY NEXT SPRING" above an old photo of Uğur and Özlem in lab coats, grinning widely,[9] and a graph of the company's share price skyrocketing. *The Economist* said the efficacy data marked "the start of the end of the pandemic."

Global media outlets also swamped BioNTech's PR team with hundreds of requests per hour. For the first time, Uğur and Özlem were interviewed together, as business partners and as husband and wife. Back in March, Uğur had balked at being profiled by a reporter, telling Jasmina Alatovic, BioNTech's comms chief, that he did not like talking about himself. Now, with a message on vaccine efficacy to communicate, he and Özlem were only too happy to speak to journalists over Zoom, from the annex that functioned as their makeshift office, with a sole plant in the background belying their newfound importance on the global stage.

Uğur would often forget to close the door behind him, leaving the family's living room exposed. "I became an expert in army-crawling across the floor," recalls the couple's daughter, who was trying to avoid being broadcast to the world. Her violin practice became impossible.

With the couple all over the news, politicians in Berlin and Brussels, with whom Helmut had been remonstrating for months, also texted their terse congratulations to the BioNTech chairman. One man, however, was still unhappy. Donald Trump, already questioning the legitimacy of the election in which he had been defeated, fired off a flurry of tweets. "As I have long said, @Pfizer and the others would only announce a Vaccine after the Election, because they didn't have the courage to do it before. Likewise, the @US_FDA should have announced it earlier, not for political purposes, but for saving lives!" he wrote.[9] He went on to allege that Democrats had deliberately delayed the efficacy data.[10] In three months, Trump would be out of the White House, but his capacity to undermine public trust in a vaccine remained a threat.

In Europe, meanwhile, political leaders found themselves in the spotlight as the public questioned why the EU had not yet procured supply of its homegrown, blockbuster vaccine. Suddenly, there was a sense of urgency in negotiations with Brussels. "As soon as they figured the horse was just about to bolt, they wanted to stop it and jump on it," says Sean Marett, BioNTech's chief commercial officer, who, alongside Pfizer counterparts, was leading the company's negotiations with the bloc.

For his part, Uğur, ever the sober scientist, was much less critical of the EU's approach. It was difficult, he says, for it to make an informed decision about a vaccine based on a novel technology, until experts were furnished with supporting data. "Our horse was quite unknown at the start of the vaccine race," he says. "The commission waited until there was evidence—it was an evidence-based strategy."

Indeed, two days after the efficacy data was publicized, on November 11, the European Union published a statement saying it was in the process of agreeing to purchase two hundred million doses, with the option to purchase one hundred million more. But the contract, signed the next day, was half the size of the one the U.S.—which has a smaller population—had placed almost four months earlier, and not all EU member states[11] were interested in the BioNTech vaccine.[12] In the end, Germany's health minister, Jens Spahn, agreed to take a much bigger chunk of the early order—roughly one hundred million doses—to swallow the shortfall caused by those countries that did not want to participate. Later, Germany returned seventy million doses[13] to the pool, fueling speculation that it was France, which was betting on its own vaccine developer, Sanofi, that had refused to participate in the first round—a claim denied by Paris.[14] "Let's just say you cannot take seventy million doses away from the pro rata because Malta was not ordering," a person familiar with the process explained.

Soon after the deal was done, the resistance in Brussels to backing the BioNTech/Pfizer vaccine was publicly confirmed by the health spokesperson for the largest group in the European Parliament. German MEP Peter Liese, who was kept abreast of negotiations, wrote that the deal took so long because, in his opinion, "there have been problems with Pfizer." "BioNTech," he wrote, "is a serious German medium-size company, whereas Pfizer is an American big company with obviously different ideas, and therefore, patience and pressure were needed in order to strike a good and fair contract." Liese, a member of Angela Merkel's Christian Democrats, went on to say that "Pfizer had ideas that were difficult to accept . . . e.g. with regards to data transparency and liability."[15]

Later, BioNTech's supervisory board was to learn that lobbyists had been employed in Brussels to urge lawmakers not to work with the company, or its American counterpart, which was labeled as "the epitome of cold capitalism." According to one person briefed on the tactics, those lobbyists argued that "if we give one euro to CureVac, or Sanofi, or a European company, it is one euro for Europe. If we give it to BioNTech, fifty cents will always end up in the U.S."

A week later, Moderna published data that showed its vaccine was nearly 94.5 percent effective,[16] cementing mRNA technology's position as the leader in the race to beat COVID-19. BioNTech and Pfizer had known since that fateful Sunday that the independent committee's interim analysis had found their vaccine to be *even more* effective, but decided to only communicate "over 90 percent" to avoid disappointment if the final analysis came up with a slightly lower figure. On November 18, BioNTech and Pfizer released that analysis, which found that of 170 individuals confirmed to have caught coronavirus, just 8 had been given two doses of the vaccine, rendering the product 95 percent effective. Crucially, efficacy was over 94 percent for those sixty-five years of age and older—the group most vulnerable to the virus, bucking the trend for vaccines against most other infectious diseases, which tend to provide less protection for the elderly. The unknowns had finally been addressed: the vaccine worked, was safe, and protected those who needed it most. The companies announced that they would apply for authorization in the UK, U.S., and EU within days, paving the way for the start of the largest vaccination campaign in human history.

The celebrations did not last long. On the same day, Germany's president, Frank-Walter Steinmeier, was interviewed by the Berlin newspaper *Tagesspiegel.*[17] "We can be proud that thanks to the admirable efforts of Özlem Türeci and Uğur Şahin and their team, a decisive contribution to overcoming the Corona pandemic will come from Germany," he said. But he implored Europe not to horde the vaccine for its own use. The bloc "should now send a political signal that they are prepared to give up part of their quota . . . to protect, for example, health workers in poorer countries of the world as quickly as possible," he wrote, in comments that were splashed on the front page.

Others fretted about what the temporary cold-chain requirements would mean for the developing world—as the BioNTech vaccine would have to be kept at roughly minus 70 degrees Celsius while being transported. "It was slightly bittersweet," says Lynda Stuart, an immunologist and director at the Bill & Melinda Gates Foundation, who had been in that Berlin hotel room in 2018 when Uğur told the billionaire that mRNA vaccines could hold the key to fighting outbreaks of infectious diseases. "Once we knew it worked, we were also faced with the logistical problem of how do we actually get this to poor and low-income countries."

For the moment, however, such concerns were moot. BioNTech was already working on stabilizing BNT162b2 so that it could be stored in regular fridges, and in the interim, COVAX, the global initiative in charge of ensuring equitable access, would prioritize procuring vaccines that presented less of a logistical challenge, such as the Oxford/AstraZeneca jab, which also looked set to be authorized by regulators around the world in a matter of weeks.

While Sean fielded calls from countries desperately trying to secure doses of the vaccine—his wife had banished him from the house due to the constant interruptions, forcing him to speak to lawmakers from his front garden—a small subset of the Lightspeed team was working day and night to prepare the paperwork for the vaccine's approval or authorization in several countries. The partnership with Pfizer proved once again to be pivotal—there was simply no way BioNTech could compile the necessary documents for a marketing authorization application on its own from scratch. The American pharma giant, which had commercialized hundreds of drugs, had a template that had been refined over several years, which could now be filled with precise data on BioNTech's production processes and safety checks. As soon as new information came in from trial sites, it was slotted in and passed on to authorities in London, Amsterdam, and Maryland, in the United States.

Unlike the FDA in America, the European Medicines Agency (EMA) was pursuing a conditional marketing authorization for the vaccine, rather than one that expired as soon as a medical emergency subsided. As a result, it wanted a more comprehensive data set, even if this took an extra couple of weeks. Individual member states could offer emergency authorizations of their own, but fell in behind the EMA, with the notable exception of Britain's MHRA. Although still officially in the European Union, the country was due to leave the bloc at the end of the year and, with a foot outside the door, wanted to hedge its bets with its own authorization process.

The MHRA, which had been accepting filings from BioNTech and Pfizer since October, urged the companies to submit clinical trial results as fast as possible and helped to speed things up. Among the last bits of data the regulator was waiting for were results from a second toxicology study, carried out on pregnant rats, to have an indication as to whether the vaccine was just as safe for those expecting children. The study—taking place in Lyon, France—was not yet complete. First, investigators had to wait for the female rats to complete their term (rat pregnancies last for around twenty-one days), before analyzing the animal subjects' organs. The final step was quality control, in which the findings would be double-checked by a second team. The UK regulator, however, agreed to accept an interim report.

On December 2, 2020, exactly ten months and eight days after Uğur first read the *Lancet* article, and just three weeks after the efficacy data came through, the MHRA became the first regulator to authorize a clinically tested COVID-19 vaccine. Simultaneously, it became the first watchdog in history to authorize an mRNA drug. Before Project Lightspeed, BioNTech had planned for an initial approval, for one of its cancer therapies, in 2023. A global tragedy had accelerated their timelines, but the team had no time to rejoice when the news came through. The moment was marked by a congratulatory page in the presentation at the next morning's virtual meeting. After a cursory "well done," Uğur clicked through to the next slide. "Now, on to today's tasks."

There was more euphoria in Britain, where politicians, including health secretary Matt Hancock, were claiming the authorization as a win for Brexit,[18] even though the UK, like other EU member states, could have diverged from the EMA's centralized plan at any point. The MHRA, keenly aware that the news would be politicized, delivered a master class in public health communications. Instead of standing alongside ministers, June Raine, the pharmacologist in charge of the agency, held a separate press conference, alongside two other independent experts who had played a role in the authorization process. Slowly and methodically, she outlined how the MHRA had implemented a "rolling review" to get a vaccine into arms "in the shortest time possible." Reading from printed notes, she added emphatically: "But, that doesn't mean any corners have been cut, none at all."[19]

On the very same morning, the EMA slightly undermined this message by suggesting that its procedure required more evidence and safety checks than Britain's emergency process.[20] It's a suggestion rejected by Constanze Blume, BioNTech's vice president of global regulatory affairs, who was working tirelessly to get information to regulators. "We only had one clinical trial," she says, "and we only had one or two manufacturing sites—how can we generate different sets of data?"

Ruben Rizzi, who worked closely with Constanze, is adamant that the speed was merely a result of a reduction in bureaucracy. "If you have everyone willing to work literally around the clock, and you have questions and responses two or three times a day that would normally require a ten- or twenty-hour turnaround—this is how you get things done," he says. "That was the kind of commitment that we had; this was the biggest shortcut."

The race to feed information to regulators overshadowed the moment in which *the Vaccine,* now universally referred to with a definite article, made history; the moment immortalized by a BNT162b2 vial in London's Science Museum, alongside the lancet used for Edward Jenner's smallpox inoculations in the eighteenth century. On December 8, Maggie Keenan, who had been among the first in Britain to receive the BCG jab in the 1950s,[21] rolled up her sleeve at a hospital in Coventry, UK, and became the first to receive a clinically authorized coronavirus shot. Live pictures of the retired jewelry shop assistant's injection were broadcast around the world, as was her message. "It's the best early birthday present I could wish for," Maggie, who would turn ninety-one in a week, told the media, "because it means I can finally look forward to spending time with my family and friends in the new year after being on my own for most of the year."[22] Her sentiments were echoed by hundreds of those who received the vaccine in the following hours, joyfully giving interviews to the global press.

Uğur and Özlem saw none of these scenes unfold. They were more than 450 miles away, at home in Mainz, plowing through documents required by European and American bodies to authorize the drug in their territories by the end of the year. "We closely followed the journey of the vials to the UK and were kept informed," says Özlem, "but we were too busy to watch the footage live." Uğur, whose quiet confidence in the success of his company's scientific quest seemed unshakable throughout the pandemic, admits he was nervous. Despite having seen the vaccine administered to more than twenty-two thousand of the forty-four thousand people in clinical studies (the rest got a placebo), he says, "It is a different feeling when people are vaccinated in the real world."

Later, however, the doctors watched the clips of Maggie and others, separately, on their smartphones. "I was touched," says Uğur. "We had always focused on individualized cancer drugs, and in that moment, I realized that even though developing an infectious disease vaccine had sometimes seemed so impersonal, there would now be billions of personal stories." For Özlem, the videos of nurses fussing over elderly patients triggered flashbacks to a similar setting: the hospital in Homburg, where she had trained as a physician and where the couple met. Having grown up watching her father care for the sick, she missed the days of working on the ward and attending to patients in person. These days, she seldom saw or heard from those who were helped by her and Uğur's innovations, but on that Tuesday evening, the beneficiaries had names, and faces, and loved ones smiling out at her from the screen. "It felt wonderful," Özlem says, "to be that close to the outcome again."

On the other side of the pond, the FDA, no longer fearing the wrath of a lame-duck president, was doing its bit to shore up public trust. The agency had taken no chances when it came to securing the data it would receive from Pfizer: it sent armed agents to the company's New York headquarters to pick up an encrypted hard drive, with a small built-in keypad and LCD display. Too many wrong attempts at entering the correct PIN code would lead to the drive being automatically deleted. But with those precautions taken, the process became radically transparent.

On Thursday, December 10, a panel of external experts held a meeting, streamed live on the internet, and clipped on rolling news channels. The committee members—connected via scratchy videoconference software from their homes—ran through a comprehensive list of safety and efficacy concerns, such as whether the vaccine should be given to people with allergies, pregnant women, or those breastfeeding babies. They discussed the thorny ethical question of whether those who received a placebo in the Phase 3 trial ought to be given the real vaccine now or be prevented from doing so while others in the general public were getting theirs. To gather data from the study on long-term side effects, there needed to be a control group that had not received the vaccine, which could be used as a comparison. But was it right to withhold a lifesaving drug from tens of thousands of people for the sake of a clean readout? The debate went back and forth, with no immediate resolution.

After more than eight hours of discussion, the chair moved on to the key question on the agenda: "Based on the totality of scientific evidence available, do the benefits of the Pfizer-BioNTech COVID-19 Vaccine outweigh its risks for use in individuals sixteen years of age and older?" The vote came in minutes later. Four panel members had voted no (two later said they wanted more data on sixteen- and seventeen-year-olds[23]), and one had abstained. Seventeen had voted yes. The next day, the FDA issued its own emergency-use authorization.

For the next few days, Uğur's and Özlem's inboxes began flowing with pictures from grateful correspondents, often families who were soon to be reunited with elderly relatives after months of painful separation. The newspapers were filled with pictures of famous people getting the jab, including President-Elect Joe Biden, who did so live on TV, and, in the UK, Ian McKellen, one of the stars of Uğur and Özlem's beloved *Lord of the Rings* movies.

The barrage of photos increased the scrutiny of the EMA, which had announced that it planned to make its decision no sooner than December 29. When its Irish head, Emer Cooke, said the agency was "working around the clock" to accelerate the process,[24] the German newspaper *Bild*—Europe's best-selling newspaper—sent photographers to its Amsterdam headquarters and splashed pictures of the building's lights being shut off at 11:00 p.m.[25] on its home page. Cooke and the agency's undoubted hard work wasn't helped by a cyberattack in which confidential filings to the EMA from BioNTech were accessed.

The company was put under pressure itself to release the millions of doses it had reserved for the EU, rather than wait until early 2021 for the bloc to start its vaccination campaign. But despite all the trials and tribulations he had gone through in negotiations, Sean resolutely refused to do so. Then, on December 21, seventy-six days after it had received the first tranche of data, the EMA approved the vaccine, shortening a process that normally takes several months. Ursula von der Leyen would later say that while the extra few weeks the EMA took to reach the decision were "crucial to trust and safety," there were "also lessons to be drawn" from the delay.[26] But the moment was marked by relief more than recrimination. Cooke hailed the approval as "an indication that 2021 can be brighter than 2020," and an initial rollout across the EU was planned for a week later.

The European Commission, meanwhile, was facing a backlash from lawmakers across the continent who wondered why it had not secured more doses for its own citizens earlier on. Markus Söder, the premier of Bavaria and a member of Angela Merkel's governing coalition, said the EU had ordered "too late and too little" and had been "stingy" in its negotiations with manufacturers.[27] Leaders in Austria, Poland, and Hungary joined the chorus of condemnation.[28] Months later, French president Emmanuel Macron would admit that the EU "didn't shoot for the stars," adding, "We didn't go fast enough, strong enough on this. We thought the vaccines would take time to take off."[29]

On January 6, 2021, Jörg Wojahn, the EU's representative in Berlin, would send a letter to the German parliament, seeking to justify the bloc's slow vaccine procurement process. "The negotiations with BioNTech took place at a time when it was not even remotely certain that the vaccine would have the necessary efficacy and would be the first preparation to be approved in 2020," he would write. "If this had been objectively evident at such an early stage, the entire world would have invested in BioNTech and production capacities for this one vaccine and the company would not have any supply problems today," he would go on to argue, not mentioning the three-quarters of a billion dollars raised by BioNTech at that juncture, from investors around the globe, in a funding round that was more than three times oversubscribed.

But in fact, cash alone may not have made the process much faster. In early February, the European Commission's vaccine negotiator, Sandra Gallina, would be hauled in front of the EU parliament's budget committee to defend her team's actions.[30] "We definitely would not have obtained more doses with more money," she would say, "because the problem . . . is manufacturing."[31] Her remarks would draw the ire of commentators, not least Nobel Prize–winning economist Paul Krugman, who called the bloc's vaccine procurement a "debacle" that would "almost surely end up causing thousands of unnecessary deaths."[32]

Yet Sierk Poetting, who was overseeing the scale-up of manufacturing, believes Gallina was right. "I think it is true," he says of her claim. "We built as fast as we could, we ramped up our lipid supply as fast as we could." While a global effort to secure the supply of raw materials may have been of some assistance, merely throwing money at the problem would not have helped. Until the company moved into its new facility at Marburg, they did not even know what equipment they would need for production, Sierk says. "If there had been two billion euros more [in funding for BioNTech], the additional manufacturing would not have been there in November." Now, the company, whose vaccine contracts are worth more than €12 billion, can afford to build more factories on its own. "Honestly," Sierk says of the effort in 2020, "there wasn't much more we could have done."

Pfizer's Albert Bourla has a similar view. He is more critical of the U.S., whose Operation Warp Speed, he says, "threw so much money that something [stuck] to the wall," referring to Moderna's successful mRNA vaccine. He does not think that the arm of the Trump administration, from which he refused to accept funding, "allocated bets in the right way," and condemns the country's attempts to restrict exports of domestically manufactured jabs to other nations until its citizens were vaccinated.[33] Europe "at least tolerated that part of the production in Europe could go to other countries," Albert says in defense of the bloc. "In the U.S., for several reasons, it was very difficult."

Whatever the relative merits of U.S. and EU approaches, in November, Brussels needed to quiet its critics by securing the optional one hundred million doses in the contract it had just signed. BioNTech and Pfizer had set aside some extra capacity for the continent, at their own risk. But in the immediate term, there would be significant bottlenecks in supply due to a complication with the production of lipid nanoparticles, the fatty wrappers that protect the vaccine's mRNA.

The problem had preoccupied Uğur in the weeks leading up to the efficacy announcement. To ensure that these crucial components were manufactured at the same quality even when produced in enormous quantities, each batch had to be individually tested and verified. But initial runs failed these tests, and no one at BioNTech or Pfizer was entirely sure why. As the vaccine plants ground to a halt, teams at both companies performed dozens of experiments to try to get to the bottom of the issue. "I was reading papers published thirty years earlier to understand the potential impact of salts and other contaminants on the testing process," says Uğur. Soon it became clear, however, that the problem lay with one of the lipids' components, produced by an external supplier. Teams at Pfizer found a way to fix this, but the remedy came too late to compensate for the lost production. Vaccine production for the last few weeks of 2020 had to be halved, from one hundred million doses, to just fifty million.

Much of that reduced capacity had already been promised to the first movers: the U.S. and the UK. President Ursula von der Leyen, however, was about to be handed a lifeline, thanks to BioNTech's relentless pursuit of additional manufacturing sites. On November 24, Sean sent an email to Sandra Gallina: "We discussed the desire of the commission to exercise its option," he wrote, knowing that with an electronic paper trail, the proposal would have to be considered. "As you know from our discussions over the summer and early autumn, the production capacity is very limited in the first half of the year." However, he added, BioNTech may have found a way through the Marburg facility to get the EU half of the one-hundred-million option in the first six months of 2021. Over the phone, he told the commission that he "needed their help" to make this happen. "We just need our production facilities approved in record time. Instead of the usual six to eight months, we need it done in three."

On December 23, an email came through confirming the additional order. Months later, the factory BioNTech had fought for, initially with no financial assistance, would help the bloc save face. The German health ministry had worked with local authorities near Marburg to get the site licensed and running by February 2021.

Four hundred staff would work at the plant, half of them in 24-7 shifts. A single batch of mRNA—which takes roughly two days to produce—would contain enough material for eight million vaccine doses. The product, made in a bioreactor named Maggie, in honor of the first person to receive the approved vaccine, would be purified and formulated before being bagged and sent to fill-and-finish sites across Europe, to be put in vials and labeled. On its way out of the building, the precious cargo would pass a glistening sign, newly installed by BioNTech's staff. It read *Aus Marburg in die Welt*—"From Marburg, into the world."

Late on Christmas Eve, Uğur and Özlem finally allowed themselves a moment of quiet pride. Uğur's professor during his sabbatical in Zurich, the seventy-six-year-old immunologist Hans Hengartner, messaged to say that he had been a beneficiary of BNT162b2 on the second day of Switzerland's vaccination program. Moments later, Roshni Bhakta, BioNTech's energetic business development director, video-called to tell him and Özlem that the company had just finalized a supply agreement with Turkey, where the couple still had elderly relatives. When Roshni asked Uğur how it felt to have developed a drug that would now help the people of his ancestral land, he paused. On his tablet, Uğur had been flicking through pictures that had just come in from Mexico, now the epicenter of the pandemic and the first nation in Latin America to begin a vaccination campaign. An initial shipment of 3,000 doses had landed in the country, where the death toll had exceeded 120,000,[34] the fourth highest total worldwide. Irene Ramírez, a fifty-nine-year-old nurse in charge of the intensive care unit at the Rubén Leñero hospital in Mexico City, which had been stretched to the breaking point, was filmed receiving the first injection, and medical staff were queuing around the block to follow suit. "Roshni," Uğur said, looking up from his screen, "it is *all* personal."

10

THE NEW NORMAL

Es gibt nichts Gutes, außer man tut es.
(Nothing good happens if one doesn't make it happen.)

—Erich Kästner

Christmas brought with it further tidings of comfort and joy in the form of pictures arriving in Uğur's and Özlem's inboxes. Christoph Prinz—the quality assurance manager at BioNTech who had overseen mRNA production—forwarded a photo of 1,600 dry ice boxes filled with vaccines at Pfizer's facility in Puurs, Belgium, ready to be shipped to countries across the EU. Others emailed images of trucks lining up at the plant to deliver the world's most precious product to distribution centers across the continent. "Many thanks for sharing," Uğur wrote in response to his team's messages. "Let me share a photo indicating the batch size with which we started." He attached a snapshot of a thumb-size plastic tube, which just over a decade earlier had contained the first strand of synthetic mRNA that he, Özlem, and their team had produced. The humble molecule was now, improbably, the basis of a medical marvel, bringing relief to a traumatized world, not to mention exhausted Lightspeed staff. "Congrats for making this possible," Uğur signed off. "Happy Holidays."

There was good news coming in from the U.S. too, where doctors and nurses were making a lifesaving discovery.[1] After thawing the frozen material in the first batches of vaccine they received from Pfizer, and diluting it with saline solution as instructed, they noticed there was enough liquid left for an extra, *sixth* dose. The scarce supply of BNT162b2, it seemed, had instantly increased by a fifth, with tens of millions more doses available to protect those most vulnerable to the pandemic.

The moment was celebrated on rolling news channels as a Christmas miracle. Yet to Uğur, it was anything but. For weeks, he had been insisting that more than five doses could be drawn from each vial. Since not all syringes are the same, and some retain a little more liquid on their walls than others, producers err on the side of caution and allow for some spillover. But with a newcomer's clarity, Uğur had pointed out to his more experienced Pfizer counterparts that there was almost enough for *seven* doses in each vial and that too much material was going to waste.

His attempts at getting them to change the recommendation on how much vaccine could be extracted, however, had been unsuccessful. Pfizer's team said it would return to the topic at a later date. Unsatisfied, Uğur asked Sierk Poetting to order millions of special "low dead volume" syringes—identified by Alex Muik, who had screened dozens of different designs—with the intention of distributing them to clinicians once this disparity was identified. Yet again, his prescience paid dividends. America's FDA advised that given the public health emergency, it was "acceptable" to use a sixth dose from each vial. The European Medicines Agency would soon follow suit, and the syringes Sierk procured would be sent to vaccination centers across the continent.

With these kinks ironed out, and the global rollout of BNT162b2 underway, Uğur and Özlem began to slowly exhale. They took a couple of days off over the new year, spent at home with their daughter. They used the full-body hazmat suits Uğur had panic-bought on Amazon eleven months earlier to clean their balcony, which had been neglected as the doctors attended to the small matter of producing the world's first clinically approved coronavirus vaccine. Suddenly, however, the family's newfound peace was shattered. Concerned friends and colleagues were getting in touch with an urgent question: Would the jab still work?

The source of the correspondents' panic was a slow-brewing news story that had started in early December, when public health officials in the UK had come across a strange data set in their weekly meeting.[2] It showed a sudden spike in infections in the county of Kent, to the southeast of London. A brief investigation soon showed there was a new variant of SARS-CoV-2 knocking about in the "Garden of England." Typically, a virus would randomly mutate a couple of times a month,[3] but this one had already managed to acquire seventeen mutations—a far greater number than experts had *ever* encountered at this stage in a pathogen's life cycle.[4] British prime minister Boris Johnson warned that the variant was 70 percent more transmissible than the original "wild type" form of the coronavirus, and some experts suggested it might be deadlier too. Within days, Britain became a pariah state, as governments banned all travel to and from the island. The controls came too late. The "Kent variant" was soon discovered in dozens of countries, from Austria to Australia.

In truth, mutations were to be expected. The version of the coronavirus that had infected tens of millions of people around the globe was *itself* slightly different from the one detected in Wuhan. The world was quickly learning one of the basic tenets of virology, which is that viruses evolve if allowed to replicate. Or as one meme circulating on social media put it: "What doesn't kill you mutates and tries again."

Nonetheless, the Kent variant scared scientists, including some of the couple's contemporaries. This time, the target of the vaccines, the spike protein protrusion, had been significantly altered.[5] Another variant was soon discovered in South Africa, which also changed the configuration of this all-important structure.

One by one, Uğur and Özlem calmed friends and colleagues. "There is too much excitement," a relaxed Uğur told an acquaintance at the time. "Every day, something must happen." Taking a break from Facebook and Twitter, he added, was to be recommended.

It was foolhardy, in the couple's view, to be alarmed about a particular variant before it had been established that it was escaping the immunity acquired by infection or by getting the vaccine. "You cannot outpace the speed of mutations," says Özlem, "and we needed a scientifically rooted understanding about whether the available vaccines failed to cross-protect against some new variant before moving ahead with a new construct." For her and Uğur, the real question was: How could the variants that might necessitate an adaptation of the vaccine be distinguished from those that would not?

The doctors had the luxury of waiting for clarity, thanks to the crucial change Uğur had insisted on back in June. While supply-chain and man-ufacturing teams were imploring BioNTech and Pfizer's management to plow ahead with the first of the Phase 1 candidates to deliver positive data—the BNT162b1—the couple had hung on until the very last minute for the delayed B2.9.

Well before they made this decision, Özlem says, it was known that the spike protein—especially its business end, the receptor-binding domain—was prone to mutations and that it might evade neutralizing antibodies over time. This was why the Lightspeed team had deliberately harnessed the combined forces of the immune system—antibodies *and* T-cells—in the first place.

If antibodies, which are trained to identify the *configuration* of virus proteins, did not properly recognize the shape-shifted spike, they would fail to disrupt the docking mechanism by which the pathogen latches onto lung cells. But T-cells—those sharpshooters the couple had spent years directing against tumors—recognize unique *features* on cells that have succumbed to infection and devour them. Most of these features, the couple understood, would be conserved across different strains (a hypothesis that was confirmed in 2021 by data from their Phase 1 trial[6]) and remain detectable for T-cells despite mutations to the spike. Thus, the particles that slipped through the first net—antibodies—would be caught by the second—T-cells—which could come to the rescue.

The successful B2.9, which encoded for the full spike protein, was able to elicit a far *broader* T-cell response than the B1, which encoded for the smaller receptor-binding domain. A *broader* immune response meant that T-cells were directed against more regions of the spike, giving them a greater chance of stopping the virus after it had invaded lung cells. "In retrospect," Özlem says, "we would not be in such a good position with regard to variants if we went with B1."

Plus, since the efficacy of the BioNTech vaccine against the original virus was so high, the company had room to maneuver. Even if a mutation of the coronavirus caused it to be 10 percent less effective, it would still provide protection to more than seventeen out of every twenty people dosed. Tests would soon prove that while the vaccine did indeed lose a few percentage points of efficacy against certain strains, it remained very potent, offering far more protection than many commonplace vaccines offered against other infectious diseases.

But there was another reason for the couple to feel confident. When questioned by reporters, Uğur explained that BioNTech had the capability to tweak its vaccine and have a variant-proof version ready for production within six weeks. The years of experience with individualized cancer vaccines, which required a unique production run for every single patient, would once again come to the fore. Manufacturing master Andreas Kuhn and his teams had gone through the cycle of analyzing genetic information; isolating a unique antigen, or vaccine target; encoding it in mRNA; and producing a finished pharmaceutical hundreds of times. A separate group[7] had been tasked with Operation Pelé—so named because Uğur wanted it to emulate the Brazilian footballer, who "built something from nothing"—whose aim was to enable the company to quickly produce commercial batches of a coronavirus vaccine and any other drugs that might be authorized in the future. The processes set in place now functioned like a well-oiled machine.

Changing the vaccine to target a new variant would not be the challenge. The essential chemistry would remain the same. The production runs would remain the same too, except for the fact that the DNA template from which the RNA is produced—that small plastic bottle with swirly liquid inside—would arrive with a slightly different sequence. Just a few of the four thousand letters in the spike protein's code would have been switched. The open question at the start of 2021 was whether regulators would allow a lightly altered candidate to proceed straight to production or require further data from clinical trials.

Meanwhile, on January 14, Uğur and Özlem went back into the office for the first time in months, where they waited in a line with employees for a doctor to administer the only BioNTech drug from which they could physically benefit. The German health ministry had prioritized the company's staff in the nationwide vaccination campaign, to ensure its vital operations were not interrupted by illness, but Uğur says he had "mixed feelings" about jumping the queue. For her part, Özlem says she was "very emotional to see the vial with BioNTech written on it. The awareness of humankind's vulnerability had felt like a burden—it suddenly seemed not as heavy anymore."

Two months later, on March 11, data from the ministry of health in Israel—the first country to have vaccinated a significant majority of its population purely with the BioNTech vaccine—lightened that load further. It showed the shot to be even more impressive in the real world than it had proved to be in clinical trials, achieving 97 percent effectiveness in preventing severe disease and death. The analysis also found the vaccine had significantly mitigated the nightmare scenario that had alarmed Uğur in January 2020, while reading the *Lancet* article. BNT162b2 was 94 percent effective at stopping *asymptomatic* spread of SARS-CoV-2.

The silent assassin had, for now, been stopped in its tracks.

On the Thursday following the release of these encouraging statistics, Uğur and Özlem boarded a train to Berlin to receive Germany's highest civilian honor, the Bundesverdienstkreuz, from the country's president, Frank-Walter Steinmeier.

The next morning, before a planned lunch with Chancellor Angela Merkel—a fellow trained scientist whom Özlem was "very excited to meet"—a grand ceremony kicked off in the presidential residence, the neoclassical Bellevue Palace. The couple—who just months earlier were unknown to all but a handful of their compatriots—were lauded by Steinmeier as two of modern Germany's greatest-ever citizens.

Uğur, uncharacteristically clad in a dark jacket and a green-striped tie, and Özlem, in a navy trouser suit, listened appreciatively as the president extolled their virtues of courage, drive, and humility. "We need these qualities in quantity in our country!" he exclaimed as the television cameras zoomed out to reveal two glistening gold medals on a table to his left.

The effusive praise was in step with much of the domestic media coverage in the wake of BioNTech's breakthrough. *Der Spiegel* magazine dubbed the duo "the German hero couple,"[8] pointing out that the country, which lags behind the U.S. when it comes to grooming successful entrepreneurs, was still brimming with ingenuity. But some of the responses focused more on Uğur's and Özlem's backgrounds than their achievements. FROM THE CHILD OF A GUEST WORKER TO A WORLD RESCUER, ran one headline in Uğur's home state of North Rhine–Westphalia,[9] which typified the tone of many others.

Steinmeier, a former foreign minister who emerged as the country's collective conscience, imparted a more nuanced message. Uğur and Özlem's success, he stressed, belonged to no one but them. "Many people have tried to claim your achievements for their own, and to attach a nationality to your work," he said. The vaccine, he went on, "is not German or Turkish, nor is it American . . . Your achievements prove that both of you are outstanding scientists."

The remarks were innocuous, but necessary. While Uğur and Özlem, both introverts, found requests for selfies on family walks a little bit much, they coped well with their newfound attention, especially the sudden excitement over the technologies to which they had devoted their lives. But they found attempts to use them as political props irksome.

For years, the couple has assiduously avoided taking sides in such debates. Helma Heinen, their long-standing assistant, says that in the run-up to elections, she would receive letters from the local branches of the conservative CDU and the center-left SPD parties, asking if they could visit Mainz's most successful start-up for a photo op. "They were always neutral," she says of the doctors' responses. "I never heard them say a bad word about any group or religion."

Of course, says Uğur, he and Özlem understand that there are people with migration backgrounds who are encouraged by their story. The couple, who acknowledge that they "tick a couple of boxes that people are interested in" are only too happy to serve as a source of inspiration to young scientists who may feel a sense of kinship. They are proud of their shared culture, which first brought them together at the university hospital in Homburg. The one constant feature in Uğur's wardrobe is a Turkish Nazar necklace, with a blue-and-white circular charm to ward off the "evil eye," and although not fluent, the couple do speak Turkish, especially when trying to communicate without their daughter understanding.

But drawing policy prescriptions from their achievements is antithetical to the way the couple see the world. "You can use us as an argument for migration, and if something is not optimal, you can use it against migration," says Uğur. Instead, he adds, "we should just focus on the facts."

When it comes to the development of the vaccine—well on its way to becoming the most commercially successful pharmaceutical in history—the facts speak for themselves. As Uğur proudly told Angela Merkel on a videoconference in January 2021, the Lightspeed team consisted of experts from over sixty countries, and more than half were women. The partnership with Pfizer, he told *The New York Times*,[10] was helped by the fact that he and Albert Bourla bonded over "their shared backgrounds as scientists and immigrants." Katalin Karikó, who came up with a modification that underpins the mRNA platform used in BNT162b2, had fled communist Hungary to the U.S. Kathrin Jansen, who pushed Pfizer to partner with BioNTech in the first place and shepherded its scientific teams through the vaccine development process, emigrated to America from Germany. Moroccan-born Moncef Slaoui's quick decision-making at the helm of Operation Warp Speed led to the first large vaccine orders. May Parsons, the nurse who injected Maggie Keenan with that first shot in Coventry, UK, under the glare of the world's TV cameras, is a proud British Filipino.[11]

There is nothing, in Uğur and Özlem's worldview, remotely surprising about the diversity of those involved in this historic effort. Their entire philosophy, in science and in life, has always been to embrace good ideas, regardless of their origin. But if there is a lesson for wider society in the meteoric rise of BioNTech (which, according to one economist, will single-handedly lift Germany's overall wealth by 0.5 percent in 2021[12]), it is less about its staff's crossing of borders and more about the entire company's transcendence of academic, scientific, and economic boundaries.

As President Steinmeier put it, "It was a long journey from research to entrepreneurship" for Uğur and Özlem, a journey seldom taken in Germany. The two doctors ventured from their wards, to the lab, to the worlds of business, technology, and education. In a culture that tends to categorize people by the subject of their research, they had refused to stop at the edges of their disciplines. The company they set up with individualized cancer therapies in mind was imbued with so much expertise that it ended up beating back the deadliest pandemic in a generation.

That is the background that matters.

Back in 2013, while Uğur, Özlem, and their team in Mainz were working on improving BioNTech's cancer vaccine candidates, former U.S. Army doctor Colonel Matt Hepburn was recruited by America's moon shot agency, DARPA, in Arlington, Virginia, and given a clear directive. His mission, he was told by his superiors, was to "take pandemics off the table." In the following years, heeding the warning signs from outbreaks of Ebola and Zika, Hepburn headed a program that challenged scientists to develop an antibody-based prophylactic and manufacture sufficient doses to stop the spread of a disease within sixty days of blood being taken from a survivor. He enlisted mRNA researchers to help—both Moderna and CureVac had been backed by DARPA.

Few thought that such a timescale was realistic[13] or indeed that mRNA-based technologies could help achieve such an ambitious goal. The lesson from the SARS and MERS epidemics was that age-old techniques, such as contact tracing, quarantine, and isolation, remained the first line of defense against a deadly pathogen. As the Singaporean epidemiologist Chew Suok Kai succinctly put it in 2007, "We cannot deny the general truth that we still continue to battle twenty-first century scourges with a nineteenth-century toolbox supplemented by a few modern scientific advances."[14] For the first eleven months of 2020, that seemed to hold true for the novel coronavirus too. DARPA's radical scheme was not ready in time to beat the COVID-19 pandemic. Hepburn ended up working for Operation Warp Speed, the U.S. government's vaccine and therapies task force, instead.

Although not endowed with the resources of the world's richest government, BioNTech's Project Lightspeed came close to achieving Hepburn's goal for him. It took just 88 days from the day Uğur established a team to work on the vaccine, to the injection of what would be the winning candidate into humans. If one counts from when the coronavirus genome was first uploaded onto the internet, on January 11, it took the Mainz-based company 105 days to respond to the greatest public health emergency in recent history. Moderna, helped by the U.S.'s National Institutes of Health, was even faster into the clinic.

It still took another 200-odd days, however, before these mRNA vaccines could be administered to the wider population—a timescale that those with an eye on the next pandemic have been seeking to shorten. "If you think about it, none of the extremely rare safety issues[15] that have emerged were detected in the Phase 3 studies for COVID-19 vaccines," says Richard Hatchett, the head of CEPI, who worked for the Obama administration and helped lead its response to the swine flu outbreak. "The most common side effects were picked up in the initial safety and immunogenicity studies, while the rare events were detected only through careful pharmacovigilance after the vaccines were released." The main information the enormous human studies provided, he argues, was whether the vaccines were effective, "and we can determine a vaccine's effectiveness after it has been released—we do this every year for influenza."

This was something the G7 would consider when its leaders met in Cornwall, UK, in June 2021, and unveiled a plan to tackle future pandemics in just a third of the time it took to respond to COVID-19. Among the suggestions in the group's eighty-four-page *100 Days Mission* report, overseen by the UK's chief scientific advisor, Sir Patrick Vallance, was the use of human challenge trials, in which a large number of volunteers are given a vaccine and then deliberately infected, to test efficacy. If the vaccine worked, it would be immediately rolled out to the general public.

Such a move was quickly dismissed by regulators in early 2020. "It was not an option, because there were no therapies for COVID-19," says the Paul Ehrlich Institute's Isabelle Bekeredjian-Ding. Since there was no way to "rescue" a participant if the virus threatened their life, a challenge trial was considered unethical. But Bekeredjian-Ding—who was in the room in February 2020 when Uğur and Özlem asked to omit, or overlap, the toxicology study on rats—has since been looking at whether the development of a vaccine could be sped up further, in a crisis, to save millions of lives.

"The problem was that COVID was not as bad—it was not great, and a lot of people died—but it was not Ebola," she says. The disease did not sufficiently scare scientists or, indeed, the public, and both groups would need to be highly alarmed to accept an expedited process that excluded a full Phase 3 trial. Even for BNT162b2, which went through every single one of the normal drug development steps, there was a public backlash against the acceleration of trials. The Paul Ehrlich Institute and other regulators had to repeatedly reassure people that no shortcuts had been taken. If a part of the sequence is skipped in the future, Bekeredjian-Ding says, "nobody is going to stand with them." When it comes to human trials, the new normal may look very much like the old.

mRNA technology has, however, opened the door for much faster vaccines. A series of "plug-and-play" platforms could be tested in advance of the next disaster and preapproved as safe. Then, when a new virus jumps from camels or bats to humans, the antigen, or target for the immune system to recognize, would be slotted into this scaffold and the pharmaceutical immediately produced for public use. Mobile manufacturing sites could be dotted around the world, ready to respond to local outbreaks with small batches of mRNA vaccines.[16] "All pandemics start as regional problems," says the NIH's Barney Graham, the man whose stabilization of the spike protein was a key innovation of the BioNTech and Moderna vaccines, and who is devoting himself to thinking about preventing further pandemics. By better biosurveillance of animal reservoirs and installing capacity for rapid vaccine production in the developing world, he and others argue, humankind could be prevented from having to face a similar catastrophe again.

Already, agencies are proposing regulations that would allow drug developers, in the event of a new outbreak, to rely on data gathered in studies using the same types of vaccine for other infectious diseases, rather than test each element again.[17] "An open question is whether phase three trials can be shortened and simplified if the product is based on a platform," said a group of regulatory experts in June 2021.[18] This, they argued, would bring the world closer to the "one hundred days" goal.

A real-world test run for this strategy began at BioNTech's headquarters soon after that G7 meeting.

Since Uğur and Özlem had told their friends not to be unduly alarmed by variants, more data had come to the fore. When it came to severe COVID-19 disease and the prevention of hospitalizations, statistics from Israel published in July showed that BNT162b2 was still incredibly effective, offering protection against those outcomes to over 90 percent of the vaccinated population. But the so-called Delta variant—now the dominant strain in many countries—seemed to have reduced the vaccine's ability to prevent infection and symptomatic disease.

It was hard to pinpoint a single cause. The most likely reason, the couple believed, was that the level of antibodies in vaccinated people had decreased in the months since they received their second dose. Those most at risk in Israel, for example, had their last injection half a year earlier. Subsequent studies were similarly difficult to parse.

To maintain broad vaccine protection, a third dose of BNT162b2 might be needed half a year after the first two, Uğur told reporters, and like with the flu, there would probably be a need for booster shots every one to two years after that. If necessary, these additional doses could be tailored to tackle rampant variants in far fewer than one hundred days. "This," Uğur said, introducing a phrase that would become commonplace once vaccine euphoria gave way to reality, "could be the new normal."[19]

To cover all bases, a BioNTech team led by Eleni Lagkadinou, a Greek clinical development specialist hired in 2020, has since launched studies to test a series of variant-focused constructs. One version substitutes the antigen, or wanted poster, of the original vaccine with the spike protein as expressed by the Alpha variant, as the mutation first discovered in Kent, UK, is now known. Another project targets the Delta strain, while a third explores the possibility of a *multivalent* vaccine, including both Delta and Alpha antigens in one product.

Andreas Kuhn's teams, which by July 2021 had already manufactured 14 grams of the new Delta construct in Mainz, continue to produce the vaccine material, which is formulated, once again, by Polymun in Austria. "It feels like déjà vu from a year ago," says Andreas, except this time, thanks to the new platform approach, regulators are unlikely to require more than clinical trials involving a couple of hundred people to check if tweaked vaccines prompt strong immune responses.

For a while to come, Uğur says, there will likely be endemic outbreaks. "We will need to carefully maintain protective measures such as widespread testing and social distancing," he predicts, "until a greater portion of the world's population is vaccinated." But the data from trials for variant-adjusted vaccines will "significantly enlarge our knowledge about vaccine protection and variants of concern," says Özlem, "and also help to inform the optimal path going forward." With procedures in place, BioNTech is able to prepare for every eventuality. "If in a few months there is an Ypsilon variant," says Eleni, "we will be ready for that as well."

If the story were to end here, BioNTech's achievements would still go down as one of the most important in medical and economic history. While many of the world's most experienced vaccine-makers, including

Merck and Sanofi, struggled, a small German company's first attempt at testing a clinically viable infectious disease vaccine proved wildly successful. At the time of writing, more than 1 billion doses of BNT162b2 have been supplied to more than one hundred countries or territories worldwide. That number is set to reach 3 billion by the end of 2021, making the vaccine the most widely distributed drug of all time. Despite their initial difficulties with the EU, BioNTech and Pfizer received a follow-up order for 1.8 billion doses from the bloc in May 2021,[20] in what will likely remain the largest pharmaceutical supply deal ever done for decades to come. The company that had half a billion euros' debt at the start of 2020 is now expecting revenues of €16 billion from vaccine contracts in 2021 alone.

For Uğur and Özlem, however, these accomplishments are mere pit stops in the ongoing race to prevent and eradicate human catastrophes. Despite being made multibillionaires, at least on paper, they continue to be lecturers at the university in Mainz and mentor Ph.D. students. At the time of writing, the doctors—still without a car or a TV—have not sold a single one of their BioNTech stocks.

Nor have their anchor shareholders, the Strüngmann twins. While coinvestors MIG divested most of their stake in BioNTech at the start of 2021, making a 4,500 percent return for the ordinary Germans and Austrians who years ago put their life savings into the fund, the Bavarian brothers are staying put. COVID-19, says Thomas Strüngmann, was a *zwischenstufe,* or intermediary stage. "For me, the dream was always to have a breakthrough in cancer therapy," the septuagenarian says. "This is what we are working for." Regulatory approval for the personalized therapies Uğur and Özlem envisioned as young lovers in the 1990s, he believes, is just a few years away.

The couple themselves are similarly optimistic. "The corona vaccine development benefitted from cancer research, and now our cancer programs will benefit from the success of our corona vaccine," says Uğur. Fifteen oncology products are currently being tested by the company in eighteen ongoing trials.

An mRNA vaccine for influenza, which still kills hundreds of thousands each year,[21] could come soon, as BioNTech and Pfizer's original collaboration is due to enter clinical trials, armed with an enormous amount of real-world safety data from the COVID-19 project. Uğur, Özlem, and their teams are already working on a vaccine for malaria—which affects more than two hundred million people a year, including young children—tackling the last of the "big three," alongside existing tuberculosis and HIV programs. A raft of other infectious diseases are on the to-do list in Mainz, some of which could be combated by swapping the wanted poster in existing vaccine constructs. In principle, so-called multivalent vaccines—already a feature of BioNTech's cancer drugs—which protect against several viral strains or several diseases at once are a possibility too.

More generally, mRNA gives BioNTech a "chance to democratize health care," Uğur says, by creating pharmaceuticals to eradicate even the most niche and intractable maladies. To take one example, the company is already testing a treatment for multiple sclerosis, which leverages the powers of the molecule to suppress, rather than induce, an immune response. MS occurs when the body malfunctions and attacks healthy cells. BioNTech's experimental vaccine against the illness sends in a wanted poster, with the *opposite* instruction to immune troops. It urges them to stand down and to better distinguish friend from foe.

Further down the road, mRNA's ability to communicate with the immune system could also be used to tackle everything from allergies to heart disease—for example, by stopping cells from dying during a cardiac arrest. "We can in principle interfere with any mechanism, once we have studied it deeply enough to understand how it works mechanistically," says Özlem, who believes the molecule could even, one day, help reverse the aging process.

BioNTech's horizons are expanding geographically as well as scientifically. In April 2021, Uğur traveled to Asia, establishing a base in Singapore, with ambitions to expand to Shanghai. Although no Phase 3 trial for the COVID-19 vaccine took place in China, due to the virus subsiding in the country, an authorization by regulators in Beijing is imminent.

In May, the U.S. government proposed waiving intellectual property patents to allow vaccine production in developing countries, a move viewed skeptically by the German government. Angela Merkel said she saw "more risk than chance"[22] in the proposal, questioning whether quality could be controlled. BioNTech's position had always been that it would build partnerships with audited vaccine manufacturers instead, and in July, the company announced it had joined forces with Cape Town's Biovac to make at least one hundred million doses of the coronavirus shot a year, exclusively for Africa. It also plans to construct a state-of-the-art factory on the continent, with the ambition to one day manufacture mRNA vaccines for malaria and tuberculosis at the facility.

There will undoubtedly be setbacks along the way. "That is just how innovation and entering unchartered terrain works," Uğur says. Investors whose attention was grabbed by Project Lightspeed may learn how long it takes to actually develop a drug in normal times. The coronavirus vaccine, however, was merely "proof of concept," Uğur adds. It was mRNA 1.0, and a new generation of more advanced platforms, including self-amplifying mRNA, is waiting in the wings. In the words of Pfizer's Phil Dormitzer, "The modRNA [the basis of the COVID-19 shot] is like a plow horse, but self-amplifying mRNA is the racehorse." Another of BioNTech's inventions, trans-amplifying mRNA, "has a huge potential," says Uğur, his eyes glistening at the prospect of another breakthrough. Because it is effective in very small doses, the platform might eventually make it possible to produce enough vaccine for the entire world within a few months.

"We believe these technologies will bring about another revolution," says Özlem, one that will give rise to a far more welcome "new normal" for those diagnosed with ailments of almost any kind.

"This," she adds, "was just the beginning."

EPILOGUE

To those of us who have never so much as seen the interior of a lab, science seems a serene discipline. While other careers depend on charisma, chance encounters, and corporate nous, the painstaking pursuit of truth, we believe, is as close to a pure meritocracy as it gets. The best ideas, buffeted by the unforgiving peer-review process, rise to the top. Personality and providence, it appears to the uninitiated, are unimportant.

This attitude is widespread. When writing this book, I found it among many of those tasked with supercharging innovation. Politicians talk of increasing funding for research, and of schemes to identify those with the most promising theses, at an early stage. Venture capitalists scour scientific journals in search of the most published and decorated. The story of BioNTech, many say, proves that more attention should be paid to those at the fringes of the medical establishment and more risk taken by those with the deepest pockets.

No one can argue with those conclusions. And yet the world's first clinically tested COVID-19 vaccine was a result of an extraordinary amount of alchemy, both in and out of the lab. The stars that aligned for BNT162b2 will never align in quite the same way again. A virus that proved amenable to vaccine-making was tackled by a company that had never taken an infectious diseases drug into the clinic. Moreover, it happened in Europe, which, although a global powerhouse in the publication of scientific papers, lags behind the U.S. when it comes to translating that expertise into approved medicines. The world's best financial forecasters could not, and did not, predict this success.

Science, it turned out, relies much more on serendipity than you might think.

When I started writing this book, I searched for *the* single breakthrough that underpinned the medical triumph that led to the BioNTech vaccine. But scientific progress does not lend itself to a linear narrative. As Özlem likes to stress, "Innovation does *not* happen at once." Independent and simultaneous discoveries are built upon, sometimes in silos, until individuals and ideas somehow merge, and human endeavor takes a giant, collective leap forward. You cannot reverse engineer this process. It is more than the sum of its parts.

The same is true of this story. Karl Popper would be amazed by the sheer amount of happenstance involved. Almost everyone I interviewed had a tale about how they were about to leave academia when a colleague or friend told them of an opportunity at BioNTech or of how they bumped into someone at a conference somewhere and were intrigued by mRNA. Many had reached dead ends in other academic areas or had fallen out with their supervisors. Some had switched from animal medicine to human, while others had started off in physics, or even business, before turning their attention to biology. Almost no one had gone from A to Z in a straight line.

However, there was one constant. It provided a clue, even in early 2020, as to where a successful vaccine, or mRNA drug, might come from. It was the character of Uğur and Özlem. Their chance meeting in the 1990s created a magnetic core, which attracted ideas and people from around the world in astonishing fashion. No amount of desk-based research or due diligence would have uncovered the extent to which their personalities were BioNTech's "secret sauce."

Finding and backing those with this je ne sais quoi, it seems to me, is the surest route to replicating the outcome of Project Lightspeed. It is people, not papers, that really makes the difference.

Uğur likes to quote from one of his favorite movies, *Batman Begins*, in which Liam Neeson's character tells Bruce Wayne: "Training is nothing, will is everything." It is no overstatement to say that it was the sheer will of two people that got us to this place.

The vaccine's key ingredient was not RNA. It was Uğur Şahin and Özlem Türeci.

APPENDIX

WHAT IS IN THE VACCINE?

Active Ingredient:

- Nucleoside-modified mRNA encoding the viral spike (S) glyco-protein of SARS-CoV-2.

Inactive Ingredients:

- Salts: Four different salts. These buffer the vaccines to stabilize the pH so that it matches the pH in our bodies.
- Lipids: Four different fatty molecules. They form a protective capsule around the RNA, aiding in its delivery and protecting it from immediate degradation.
- Sugar, or Sucrose: This is a *cryoprotectant*. It ensures the lipids do not get too sticky at cold storage temperatures.

WHAT IS NOT IN THE VACCINE

- Eggs, gelatin, latex, preservatives, metals, microelectronics, electrodes, carbon nanotubes, or nanowire semiconductors.[1]

ACKNOWLEDGMENTS

I would be lying if I said that I knew, in early 2020, that a small biotech twenty miles to the west of my home in Frankfurt was primed to produce the world's first and best coronavirus vaccine. In fact, I had hardly heard of BioNTech before I received an email from the *FT*'s science editor, Clive Cookson—one of the nicest people in journalism—encouraging me to speak to the company. The very next day, I was introduced to Uğur, who patiently explained mRNA and its promise. I was in no position to judge whether the technology was ripe enough and whether BioNTech had an edge over its competitors. But something about the ease with which Uğur was able to communicate the concepts underpinning his and Özlem's ambition—to develop a drug against the then far-off SARS-CoV-2 by the end of the year—made me think that here was a story worth telling, however it ended. I thank "whatever gods may be" for that instinct.

Beyond my divine gratitude, I am indebted to several people who supported me in telling this extraordinary story. Among them are John Mervin, for the invaluable advice, as well as Kim Gittleson, Claire Jones, Adam Taub, Kent De Pinto, and Josh Spero for their pep talks and free workshopping seminars.

Sam Katz, one of the NIH's most brilliant scientists, helped me understand what an assay was, and much more besides. Joseph Schneck, a walking advert for autodidacticism, gave me a crash course in biology. Geoff Dyer and Murray Withers made my first *Financial Times* "Big Read" on BioNTech sing. Martin Arnold, Olaf Storbeck, and Alexander

Vladkov, my *FT* colleagues in Frankfurt, stood watch over my beat while I attempted to put pen to paper. Several others at the *FT*, among them Peter Campbell, Erika Solomon, Hannah Kuchler, Donato Mancini, Claire Bushey, Alec Russell, Patrick Jenkins, and Tom Braithwaite, were encouraging, helpful, and most of all, patient.

Thanks also to Esther Marshall, Daniel Grabiner, Léo Gallier, Peter Littger, Simon Warner, Mike Stemke, and Julian Dillmann for keeping me sane. To Richard Hatchett for helping me map my thoughts. To all my publishers, especially Harry Scoble at Audible, George Witte at St. Martin's, Moritz Schuller and Johanna Langmaack at Rowohlt, and Ajda Vucicevic at Welbeck, for their faith and forbearance. To Jonny Geller and Viola Hayden at Curtis Brown for having my back from day one and clearing every obstacle all the way to the finish line. To Jack Ramm for getting in the trenches with me, even when running a fever, and making sure this book was as good as it could be, despite the time pressures. Without him, I would probably still be staring at some rough drafts.

To Beatrice Goldenthal and her surgery staff in Offenbach for giving me (and thousands of others) "the Vaccine." To Jan Grant, who started me on this journey back in 2008, and to the late Claire Prosser, for giving me the opportunity of a lifetime four years later.

Last but not least, thank you to all the scientists, researchers, and managers at BioNTech and beyond, who were exceedingly generous with their time, and polite enough not to ridicule my ignorance. To Jasmina Alatovic for supporting me in telling this story, independently, at every step. And of course, to Uğur and Özlem, protagonists who would be a boon to any writer, but who gave me the added gift of a free education in science and, most important, in life.

Loving thanks to Anna Noryskiewicz, who bounced into a restaurant in Berlin on a summer evening years ago and, in an instant, changed my life for the better. Without you, none of this would be possible. *Dzięki, kochanie.*

NOTES

PROLOGUE: THE COVENTRY MIRACLE

1. "Meet the nurse who gave world's first COVID-19 vaccine," *Royal College of Nursing Bulletin*, December 2020. Available at https://www.rcn.org.uk /magazines/bulletin/2020/dec/may-parsons-nurse-first-vaccine-covid-19.

2. "Landmark Moment As First NHS Patient Receives Covid-19 Vaccination at UHCW University," Hospitals Coventry and Warwickshire NHS Trust, December 2020. Available at https://www.uhcw.nhs.uk/news/landmark-moment -as-first-nhs-patient-receives-covid-19-vaccination-at-uhcw/.

3. McEnroe, Natasha, "Covid vaccine to go on display," Science Museum Group, December 2020. Available at https://www.sciencemuseumgroup.org.uk/blog /covid-vaccine-to-go-on-display/.

4. Lo, Andrew W and Siah, Kien Wei and Wong, Chi Heem, "Estimating Probabilities of Success of Vaccine and Other Anti-Infective Therapeutic Development Programs," National Bureau of Economic Research, May 2020. Available at https:// abcnews.go.com/Health/health-experts-warn-life-saving-coronavirus-vaccine- years/story?id=69032902.

5. Cannon, Kelly, "Health experts warn life-saving coronavirus vaccine still years away," ABC News, February 2020. Available at https://abcnews.go.com/Health/ health-experts-warn-life-saving-coronavirus-vaccine-years/story?id=69032902.

CHAPTER 1: THE OUTBREAK

1. Leuty, Ron, "Biotech's big JPM Healthcare Conference will go virtual in January," *San Francisco Business Times*, September 2020. Available at https://www .bizjournals.com/sanfrancisco/news/2020/09/10/jpm21-jpmorgan-healthcare -conference-virtual-jpm.html.

2. Cherry, James, and Krogstad, Paul, "SARS: The First Pandemic of the 21st Century," *Pediatric Research*, July 2004. Available at https://doi.org/10.1203/01.PDR.0000129184.87042.FC.

3. Tatem, A.J. and Rogers, D.J. et al, "Global Transport Networks and Infectious Disease Spread," *Advances in Parasitology*, April 2006. Available at https://doi.org/10.1016/S0065-308X(05)62009-X.

4. "Summary of probable SARS cases with onset of illness from 1 November 2002 to 31 July 2003," World Health Organization, July 2015. Available at https://www.who.int/publications/m/item/summary-of-probable-sars-cases-with-onset-of-illness-from-1-november-2002-to-31-july-2003.

5. "Middle East respiratory syndrome coronavirus (MERS-CoV)," World Health Organization. Available at https://www.who.int/health-topics/middle-east-respiratory-syndrome-coronavirus-mers#tab=tab_1.

6. "Mainzer Unimedizin bereitet sich auf Coronavirus vor," t-online, January 2020. Available at https://www.t-online.de/region/mainz/news/id_87212460/mainz-uni medizin-bereitet-sich-auf-coronavirus-vor.html.

7. "Frankfurt Airport Air Traffic Statistics 2019," Fraport, 2019. Available at https://www.fraport.com/content/dam/fraport-company/documents/investoren/eng/aviation-statistics/Air_Traffic_Statistics_2019.pdf/_jcr_content/renditions/original.media_file.download_attachment.file/Air_Traffic_Statistics_2019.pdf.

8. Fox, Maggie, "Kids will need two doses of H1N1 flu vaccine," Reuters, November 2009. Available at https://www.reuters.com/article/us-flu-vaccine-usa/kids-will-need-two-doses-of-h1n1-flu-vaccine-idUSTRE5A14UK20091103.

9. Borse, Rebekah and Shrestha, Sundar et al, "Effects of Vaccine Program against Pandemic Influenza A(H1N1) Virus, United States, 2009–2010," *Emerging Infectious Diseases*, March 2013. Available at https://doi.org/10.3201/eid1903.120394.

10. "Meine Eltern standen jeden Tag um 4.30 Uhr auf," *Bild*, December 2020. Available at https://www.bild.de/video/clip/news/biontech-chef-hat-tuerkische-wurzeln-meine-eltern-standen-jeden-tag-um-4-30-uhr-74570942-74572298.bild.html.

11. Ebel, Bastian, "Stolz an Kölner Schule Irrer Lebensweg: Ex-Abiturient wird in Corona-Zeit zum Weltstar," *Express*, November 2020. Available at https://www.express.de/koeln/stolz-an-koelner-schule-irrer-lebensweg—ex-abiturient-wird-in-corona-zeit-zum-weltstar-37600434?cb=1616447564414.

12. Boczkowski, David, "The RNAissance Period," *Discover Medicine*, August 2016. Available at https://www.discoverymedicine.com/David-Boczkowski/2016/08/the-rnaissance-period/.

13. Cobb, Matthew, "Who discovered messenger RNA?," *Current Biology*, June 2015. Available at https://doi.org/10.1016/j.cub.2015.05.032.

14. "World Health Summit 2018," World Health Summit, October 2018. Available at https://www.worldhealthsummit.org/about/history/2018.html.

15. "Innovation to Address Global Health and Development: Achieving the Sustainable Development Goals," YouTube, October 2018. Available at https://www.youtube.com/watch?v=s4CMQJ75FWs&t=282s.

16. Bosch, Berend and Zee, Ruurd van der and Haan, Cornelis de and Rottier, Peter, "The Coronavirus Spike Protein Is a Class I Virus Fusion Protein: Structural and Functional Characterization of the Fusion Core Complex," *Journal of Virology*, December 2020. Available at https://doi.org/10.1128/JVI.77.16.8801-8811.2003.

17. Dallmus, Alexander, "Die Ärztin, auf die keiner hörte," *Tagesschau*, January 2021. Available at https://www.tagesschau.de/inland/gesellschaft/rothe-coronavirus-101.html.

CHAPTER 2: PROJECT LIGHTSPEED

1. Blackburn, Simon, *Oxford Dictionary of Philosophy*, 2008.

2. Bewarder, Manuel and Dowldelt, Anette and Naber, Ibrahim, "Die verlorenen Wochen," *Welt*, May 2020. Available at https://www.welt.de/politik/deutschland/plus208030405/Coronakrise-78-Tage-bis-zum-Lockdown-Die-verlorenen-Wochen.html.

3. "Tagesschau 20 Uhr," *Tagesschau*, January 2020. Available at https://www.tagesschau.de/multimedia/sendung/ts-35365.html.

4. Leung, Hillary and Godin, Mélissa, "A 36-Year-Old Man Is the Youngest Fatality of the Wuhan Coronavirus Outbreak So Far," *Time*, January 2020. Available at https://time.com/5770924/wuhan-coronavirus-youngest-death/.

5. VanBlargan, Laura and Goo, Leslie and Pierson, Theodore, "Deconstructing the Antiviral Neutralizing-Antibody Response: Implications for Vaccine Development and Immunity," *Microbiology and Molecular Biology Reviews*, October 2016. Available at https://doi.org/10.1128/MMBR.00024-15.

6. Hinz, Thomas and Kallen, Kajo and Şahin, Uğur and Türeci, Özlem et al, "The European Regulatory Environment of RNA-Based Vaccines," *Methods in Molecular Biology*, December 2016. Available at https://doi.org/10.1007/978-1-4939-6481-9_13; Britten, Cedrik M. and Singh-Jasuja, Harpreet and Şahin, Uğur et al, "The regulatory landscape for actively personalized cancer immunotherapies," *Nature Biotechnology*, October 2013. Available at https://doi.org/10.1038/nbt.2708.

7. "Let's talk about lipid nanoparticles," *Nature Reviews Materials*, February 2021. Available at https://doi.org/10.1038/s41578-021-00281-4.

8. Kranz, Lena M and Diken, Mustafa and Türeci, Özlem and Şahin, Uğur et al, "Systemic RNA delivery to dendritic cells exploits antiviral defence for

cancer immunotherapy," *Nature*, June 2016. Available at https://doi.org/10.1038/nature18300.

9. Nichols, Eve, "Expanding Access to Investigational Therapies for HIV Infection and AIDS," Institute of Medicine (U.S.) Roundtable for the Development of Drugs and Vaccines Against AIDS, March 1990. Available at https://www.ncbi.nlm.nih.gov/books/NBK234129/.

10. Ibid.

11. Mende, Annette, "Vorsicht geht über alles," *Pharmazeutische Zeitung*, February 2016. Available at https://www.pharmazeutische-zeitung.de/ausgabe-052016/vorsicht-geht-ueber-alles/.

12. Stobbart, L. and Murtagh, M.J. et al, "We saw human guinea pigs explode," *British Medical Journal*, March 2007. Available at https://doi.org/10.1136/bmj.39150.488264.47.

13. "Man who died in French drug trial had 'unprecedented' reaction, say experts," *The Guardian*, March 2016. Available at https://www.theguardian.com/science/2016/mar/07/french-drug-trial-man-dead-expert-report-unprecidented-reaction.

14. Borse, Rebekah and Shrestha, Sundar et al, "Effects of Vaccine Program against Pandemic Influenza A(H1N1) Virus, United States, 2009–2010," *Emerging Infectious Diseases*, March 2013. Available at https://doi.org/10.3201/eid1903.120394.

CHAPTER 3: THE UNKNOWNS

1. Enserink, Martin, "Update: 'A bit chaotic.' Christening of new coronavirus and its disease name create confusion," *Science*, February 2020. Available at https://www.sciencemag.org/news/2020/02/bit-chaotic-christening-new-coronavirus-and-its-disease-name-create-confusion.

2. "Coronavirus disease 2019 (COVID-19) Situation Report—23," World Health Organization, February 2020. Available at https://www.who.int/docs/default-source/coronaviruse/situation-reports/20200212-sitrep-23-ncov.pdf?sfvrsn=41e9fb78_4.

3. "Novel Coronavirus(2019-nCoV) Situation Report – 12," World Health Organization, February 2020. Available at https://www.who.int/docs/default-source/coronaviruse/situation-reports/20200201-sitrep-12-ncov.pdf?sfvrsn=273c5d35_2.

4. "Corona-Virus: Bundesregierung hält Risiko für Deutschland sehr gering," *Die Rheinpfalz*, January 2020. Available at https://www.rheinpfalz.de/panorama_artikel,-corona-virus-bundesregierung-h%C3%A4lt-risiko-f%C3%BCr-deutschland-sehr-gering-_arid,1579340.html.

5. "Coronavirus: German health minister calls on EU to allocate funds," *DW*, February 2020. Available at https://www.dw.com/en/coronavirus-german-health -minister-calls-on-eu-to-allocate-funds/a-52355832.

6. VanBlargan, Laura and Goo, Leslie and Pierson, Theodore, "Deconstructing the Antiviral Neutralizing-Antibody Response: Implications for Vaccine Development and Immunity," *Microbiology and Molecular Biology Reviews*, October 2016. Available at https://doi.org/10.1128/MMBR.00024-15.

7. Randal, Judith, "Hepatitis C Vaccine Hampered by Viral Complexity, Many Technical Restraints," *Journal of the National Cancer Institute*, June 1999. Available at https://doi.org/10.1093/jnci/91.11.906.

8. Riddle, M.S. and Chen, W. et al, "Update on vaccines for enteric pathogens," *Clinical Microbiology and Infection*, October 2018. Available at https://doi.org /10.1016/j.cmi.2018.06.023.

9. Stanway, David and Kelland, Kate, "Explainer: Coronavirus reappears in discharged patients, raising questions in containment fight," Reuters, February 2020. Available at https://www.reuters.com/article/us-china-health-reinfection -explainer-idUSKCN20M124.

10. "Hong Kong reports 'first case' of virus reinfection," BBC, August 2020. Available at https://www.bbc.com/news/health-53889823.

11. Graham, Barney and Modjarrad, Kayvon and McLellan, Jason, "Novel Antigens for RSV Vaccines," *Current Opinion in Immunology*, August 2015. Available at https://doi.org/10.1016/j.coi.2015.04.005.

12. Harding, Anne, "Research shows why 1960s RSV shot sickened children," Reuters, December 2008. Available at https://www.reuters.com/article/us-rsv-shot -idUSTRE4BM4SH20081223.

13. Delgado, Maria Florencia and Coviello, Silvina et al, "Lack of antibody affinity maturation due to poor Toll-like receptor stimulation leads to enhanced respiratory syncytial virus disease," *Nature Medicine*, December 2008. Available at https://doi.org/10.1038/nm.1894.

14. Amanat, Fatima and Krammer, Florian, "SARS-CoV-2 Vaccines: Status Report," *Immunity*, April 2020. Available at https://doi.org/10.1016/j.immuni.2020.03.007.

15. Czub, Markus and Weingartl, Hana et al, "Evaluation of modified vaccinia virus Ankara based recombinant SARS vaccine in ferrets," *Vaccine*, March 2005. Available at https://doi.org/10.1016/j.vaccine.2005.01.033.

16. Liu, Li and Wei, Qiang et al, "Anti-spike IgG causes severe acute lung injury by skewing macrophage responses during acute SARS-CoV infection," *JCI Insight*, February 2019. Available at https://doi.org/10.1172/jci.insight.123158.

17. Smatti, Maria K and Thani, Asmaa A Al and Yassine, Hadi M, "Viral-Induced Enhanced Disease Illness," *Frontiers in Microbiology*, December 2018. Available at https://doi.org/10.3389/fmicb.2018.02991.

18. Ibid.

19. Cai, Yongfei, "Distinct conformational states of SARS-CoV-2 spike protein," *Science*, September 2020. Available at https://doi.org/10.1126/science.abd4251.

20. Coontz, Robert, "Science's Top 10 Breakthroughs of 2013," *Science*, December 2013. Available at https://www.sciencemag.org/news/2013/12/sciences-top-10-breakthroughs-2013.

21. Kramer, Jillian, "They spent 12 years solving a puzzle. It yielded the first COVID-19 vaccines," *National Geographic*, December 2020. Available at https://www.nationalgeographic.com/science/article/these-scientists-spent-twelve-years-solving-puzzle-yielded-coronavirus-vaccines.

22. Graham, Barney and McLellan, Jason et al, "Prefusion Coronavirus Spike Proteins and their Use," World Intellectual Property Organisation, May 2018. Available at https://patentimages.storage.googleapis.com/68/47/0c/2b5bc4f43c9f74/WO2018081318A1.pdf.

23. Highfield, Roger, "Coronavirus: the Spike," Science Museum Group, November 2020. Available at https://www.sciencemuseumgroup.org.uk/blog/coronavirus-the-spike/.

24. Gilbert, Sarah C, "T-cell-inducing vaccines – what's the future," *Immunology*, January 2012. Available at https://doi.org/10.1111/j.1365-2567.2011.03517.x.

25. Zhao, Zhongyi and Wei, Yinhao and Tao, Chuanmin, "An enlightening role for cytokine storm in coronavirus infection," *Clinical Immunology*, January 2012. Available at https://dx.doi.org/10.1016%2Fj.clim.2020.108615.

26. Ettel, Anja and Turzer, Caroline, "So gut ist Deutschland auf eine Epidemie vorbereitet," *Welt*, January 2020. Available at https://www.welt.de/wirtschaft/article205424021/Coronavirus-Behoerden-bereiten-sich-auf-hunderte-Infizierte-vor.html.

27. Giuffrida, Angela and Cochrane, Lauren, "Italy imposes draconian rules to stop spread of coronavirus," *The Guardian*, February 2020. Available at https://www.theguardian.com/world/2020/feb/23/italy-draconian-measures-effort-halt-coronavirus-outbreak-spread.

28. Jones, Sam and Burgen, Stephen and Boseley, Sarah, "Tenerife coronavirus: 1,000 guests at hotel quarantined," *The Guardian*, February 2020. Available at https://www.theguardian.com/world/2020/feb/25/tenerife-coronavirus-guests-hotel-quarantined.

CHAPTER 4: THE mRNA BIOHACKERS

1. "Regionalzug gestoppt: Coronavirus-Verdacht," *Süddeutsche Zeitung*, February 2020. Available at https://www.sueddeutsche.de/wirtschaft/bahn-idar-oberstein-regionalzug-gestoppt-coronavirus-verdacht-dpa.urn-newsml-dpa-com-20090101-200226-99-87325.

2. "Bundesregierung schickt weitere Hilfslieferung nach China," Die Zeit, February 2020. Available at https://www.zeit.de/wissen/gesundheit/2020-02/coronavirus-china-deutschland-hilfslieferung-bundesregierung-epidemie-desinfektionsmittel-schutzkleidung.

3. Hennig, Korinna and Drosten, Christian, "Coronavirus Update," NDR, February 2020. Available at https://www.ndr.de/nachrichten/info/coronaskript102.pdf.

4. Hennig, Korinna and Drosten, Christian, "Coronavirus Update," NDR, February 2020. Available at https://www.ndr.de/nachrichten/info/coronaskript100.pdf.

5. Kevles, Bettyann, "BOOK REVIEW : The Human Adventures in Ages-Old Wars Against Viruses," *Los Angeles Times*, January 1991. Available at https://www.latimes.com/archives/la-xpm-1991-01-01-vw-7522-story.html.

6. Spinney, Laura, "Smallpox and other viruses plagued humans much earlier than suspected," *Nature*, July 2020. Available at https://www.nature.com/articles/d41586-020-02083-0.

7. Barone, Paul and Wiebe, Michael et al, "Viral contamination in biologic manufacture and implications for emerging therapies," *Nature Biotechnology*, April 2020. Available at https://www.nature.com/articles/s41587-020-0507-2.

8. Yeung, Jessie, "The US keeps millions of chickens in secret farms to make flu vaccines. But their eggs won't work for coronavirus," CNN, March 2020. Available a https://edition.cnn.com/2020/03/27/health/chicken-egg-flu-vaccine-intl-hnk-scli/index.hml.

9. "Weekly 2009 H1N1 Flu Media Briefing," CDC, October 2009. Available at https://www.cdc.gov/media/transcripts/2009/t091023.htm.

10. Bender, Eric, "Accelerating flu protection," *Nature*, September, 2019. Available at https://www.nature.com/articles/d41586-019-02756-5.

11. "The innate and adaptive immune systems," Informed Health, July 2020. Available at https://www.ncbi.nlm.nih.gov/books/NBK279396/.

12. Nussenzweig, Michel, "Ralph Steinman and the Discovery of Dendritic Cells," *Nobel Prize*, December 2011. Available at https://www.nobelprize.org/uploads/2018/06/steinman_lecture.pdf.

13. Boczkowski, David, "The RNAissance Period," *Discovery Medicine*, August 2016. Available at https://www.discoverymedicine.com/David-Boczkowski/2016/08/the-rnaissance-period/.

14. "Goodbye, Dear Friend: Dr Jon Wolff," School of Medicine and Public Health, July 2020. Available at https://www.med.wisc.edu/quarterly/volume-22-number-2/goodbye-dear-friend-dr-jon-wolff/.

15. Wolff, Jon and Malone, Robert et al, "Direct Gene Transfer into Mouse Muscle in Vivo," *Science*, March 1990. Available at https://doi.org/10.1126/science.1690918.

16. Martinon, Frédéric and Krishnan, Sivadasan et al, "Induction of virus-specific cytotoxic T lymphocytes in vivo by liposome-entrapped mRNA," *European Journal of Immunology*, July 1993. Available at https://doi.org/10.1002/eji.1830230749.

17. Schijns, V.E.J.C., "Chapter 1—Vaccine Adjuvants' Mode of Action: Unraveling "the Immunologist's Dirty Little Secret," *Immunopotentiators in Modern Vaccines* (2nd ed.), 2017. Available at https://doi.org/10.1016/B978-0-12-804019-5.00001-3.

18. Lemaitre, Bruno and Nicolas, Emmanuelle et al, "The Dorsoventral Regulatory Gene Cassette spätzle/Toll/cactus Controls the Potent Antifungal Response in Drosophila Adults," *Cell*, September 1996. Available at https://doi.org/10.1016/s0092-8674(00)80172-5.

19. Poltorak, Alexander and He, Xiaolong et al, "Defective LPS Signaling in C3H/HeJ and C57BL/10ScCr Mice: Mutations in Tlr4 Gene," *Science*, December 1998. Available at https://doi.org/10.1126/science.282.5396.2085.

20. Medzhitov, Ruslan and Preston-Hurlburt, Paula and Janeway Jr, Charles, "A human homologue of the Drosophila Toll protein signals activation of adaptive immunity," *Nature*, July 1997. Available at https://www.nature.com/articles/41131.

21. Schijns, V.E.J.C., "Chapter 1—Vaccine Adjuvants' Mode of Action: Unraveling "the Immunologist's Dirty Little Secret," Immunopotentiators in Modern Vaccines (2nd ed.), 2017. Available at https://doi.org/10.1016/B978-0-12-804019-5.00001-3.

22. Enard, David and Petrov, Dmitri, "Ancient RNA virus epidemics through the lens of recent adaptation in human genomes," Philosophical Transactions of the Royal Society B, October, 2020. Available at https://doi.org/10.1098/rstb.2019.0575 .

23. Key, Lindsay, "Prepping for a Pandemic: Duke's Long History of RNA-based Vaccine Development," *Magnify*, September 2020. Available at https://medschool.duke.edu/about-us/news-and-communications/som-magnify/prepping-pandemic-duke%E2%80%99s-long-history-rna-based-vaccine-development.

24. Boczkowski, David and Nair, Smita et al, "Dendritic Cells Pulsed with RNA are Potent Antigen-presenting Cells In Vitro and In Vivo," *Journal of Experimental Medicine*, August 1996. Available at https://doi.org/10.1084/jem.184.2.465.

25. Led by Hans Hengartner, who had deciphered some of the killing mechanisms

used by T-cells, and Rolf Zinkernagel, a Nobel Prize winner who had uncovered how the immune system recognises virus-infected cells.

26. Diken, M. and Kreiter, S. and Türeci, Özlem and Şahin, Uğur et al, "Selective uptake of naked vaccine RNA by dendritic cells is driven by macropinocytosis and abrogated upon DC maturation," *Gene Therapy*, March 2011. Available at https://www.nature.com/articles/gt201117.

27. Gasser, Barbara, "Biontech-Vize Katalin Karikó "Mutter" der Corona-Impfstoffe: 'Eine Milliarde Dollar, das würde mir nur Kopfschmerzen bereiten'," *Kleine Zeitung*, April 2021. Available at https://www.kleinezeitung.at/lebensart /5960692/BiontechVize-Katalin-Kariko_Mutter-der-CoronaImpfstoffe_Eine.

28. Kranz, Lena and Diken, Mustafa and Türeci, Özlem and Şahin, Uğur et al, "Systemic RNA delivery to dendritic cells exploits antiviral defence for cancer immunother- apy," *Nature*, June 2016. Available at https://www.nature.com/articles/nature18300.

29. Ibid.

30. DeFrancesco, Laura, "The 'anti-hype' vaccine," *Nature Biotechnology*, February 2017. Available at https://www.nature.com/articles/nbt.3812#Sec1.

31. "Pocket Program," *Fourth International Cancer Immunotherapy Conference: Translating Science into Survival*, October 2018. Available at https://www.aacr .org/wp-content/uploads/2020/01/CRI18_Program-1.pdf.

32. "Press release: The Nobel Prize in Physiology or Medicine 2018," *The Nobel Prize*, October 2018. Available at https://www.nobelprize.org/prizes/medicine /2018/press-release/.

33. Şahin, Uğur and Oehm, Petra and Türeci, Özlem et al, "An RNA vaccine drives immunity in checkpoint-inhibitor-treated melanoma," *Nature*, July 2020. Avail- able at https://doi.org/10.1038/s41586-020-2537-9.

CHAPTER 5: THE TESTS

1. "BioNTech and the University of Pennsylvania Enter into Strategic Research Collaboration to Develop mRNA Vaccine Candidates Against Various Infectious Diseases," November 2018. Available at https://biontech.de/sites/default/files /2019-08/20181104_20181105_BioNTech-and-the-University-of-Pennsylvania .pdf.

2. Originally, to deliver mRNA encoded antibodies.

3. Codeveloped with Uğur and Özlem's academic group at TRON, headed by Ger- man molecular biologist Tim Beissert.

4. The team consisted of a mixture of seasoned experts with decades of mRNA expe- rience such as Uğur and Özlem, Katalin Karikó, Andreas Kuhn, Mustafa Diken, Tim Beissert, as well as young scientists, technicians, and graduate students.

5. "Coronavirus disease 2019 (COVID-19) Situation Report—40," World Health Organization, February 2020. Available at https://www.who.int/docs/default -source/coronaviruse/situation-reports/20200229-sitrep-40-covid-19.pdf ?sfvrsn=849d0665_2.

6. "Basic Laboratory Design for Biosafety Level 3 Laboratories," Oregon State University. Available at https://fa.oregonstate.edu/cpd-standards/appendix/room -and-space-types/basic-laboratory-design-biosafety-level-3-laboratories.

7. Zhang, Yuanyuan and Zhang, Zemin, "The history and advances in cancer immunotherapy: understanding the characteristics of tumor-infiltrating immune cells and their therapeutic implications," *Cellular & Molecular Immunology,* July 2020. Available at https://www.nature.com/articles/s41423-020-0488-6.

8. "Daily Situation Report of the Robert Koch Institute," March 2020. Available at https://www.rki.de/DE/Content/InfAZ/N/Neuartiges_Coronavirus /Situationsberichte/2020-03-14-en.pdf?__blob=publicationFile.

9. Merkel, Angela, "Dies ist eine historische Aufgabe - und sie ist nur gemeinsam zu bewältigen," *Die Bundesregierung,* March 2020. Available at https://www. bundesregierung.de/breg-de/themen/coronavirus/-this-is-a-historic-task-and- it-can-only-be-mastered-if-we-face-it-together--1732476.

CHAPTER 6: FORGING ALLIANCES

1. "Eli Lilly and BioNTech announce Research Collaboration," BioNTech, May 2015. Available at https://investors.biontech.de/news-releases/news-release -details/eli-lilly-and-biontech-announce-research-collaboration.

2. "BioNTech," Cipherbio. Available at https://www.cipherbio.com/data-viz /organization/BioNTech/funding.

3. EY Biotechnologie-Report, 2020.

4. Spalding, Rebecca, "Biotechnology firm ADC pulls listing amid latest IPO market jitters," Reuters, October 2019. Available at https://www.reuters.com/article /us-usa-ipo-idUSKBN1WI00R.

5. "United States Securities and Exchange Commission: Form F-1 Registration Statement," BioNTech, June 2019. Available at https://investors.biontech.de /node/7291/html.

6. "DARPA Awards Moderna Therapeutics a Grant for up to $25 Million to Develop Messenger RNA Therapeutics," Moderna, October 2013. Available at https://investors.modernatx.com/news-releases/news-release-details/darpa -awards-moderna-therapeutics-grant-25-million-develop.

7. Debolt, David, "29 people had flu-like symptoms when they died in Santa Clara County. Nine tested positive for coronavirus," *Mercury News,* April 2020.

Available at https://www.mercurynews.com/2020/04/25/9-santa-clara-deaths -reclassified-as-covid-19-related/.

8. "Coronavirus disease 2019 (COVID-19) Situation Report – 43," World Health Organization, March 2020. Available athttps://www.who.int/docs/default -source/coronaviruse/situation-reports/20200303-sitrep-43-covid-19.pdf?sfvrsn =76e425ed_2.

9. "Mission Possible: The Race for a Vaccine," YouTube, April 2021. Available at https://www.youtube.com/watch?v=jbZUZ9JYNBE.

10. "Coronavirus: German, US companies sign deal to develop vaccine," DW, March 2020. Available at https://www.dw.com/en/coronavirus-german-us-companies -sign-deal-to-develop-vaccine/a-52802822.

11. Cookson, Clive, "Fosun and BioNTech launch $135m vaccine hunt for corona-virus," *Financial Times*, March 2020. Available at https://www.ft.com/content /271ee270-6796-11ea-800d-da70cff6e4d3.

CHAPTER 7: FIRST IN HUMAN

1. "Guidelines on the Quality, Safety and Efficacy of Ebola Vaccines," World Health Organization, October 2017. Available at https://www.who.int/biologicals /expert_committee/BS2327_Ebola_Vaccines_Guidelines.pdf.

2. "Merkel announces strict measures, tells Germans to stay home in virus fight," France 24, March 2020. Available at https://www.france24.com/en/20200317-merkel -announces-strict-measures-and-tells-germans-to-stay-home-in-virus-fight.

3. "Der Proband - Ein Mannheimer lässt einen CoronaImpfstoff an sich testen," SWR 2, February 2020. Available at https://www.swr.de/swr2/leben-und -gesellschaft/der-proband-ein-mannheimer-laesst-einen-corona-impfstoff-an -sich-testen-swr2-leben-2021-02-04-102.pdf.

4. Feuer, Alan and Salcedo, Andrea, "New York City Deploys 45 Mobile Morgues as Virus Strains Funeral Homes," *New York Times*, April 2020. Available at https:// www.nytimes.com/2020/04/02/nyregion/coronavirus-new-york-bodies.html.

5. Slotnik, Daniel, "Up to a tenth of New York City's coronavirus dead may be buried in a potter's field," *New York Times*, March 2021. Available at https://www.nytimes .com/2021/03/25/nyregion/hart-island-mass-graves-coronavirus.html.

6. "Mission Possible: The Race for a Vaccine," YouTube, April 2021. Available at https://www.youtube.com/watch?v=jbZUZ9JYNBE.

7. "First Clinical Trial of a COVID-19 Vaccine Authorised in Germany," Paul-Ehrlich-Institut, August 2020. Available at https://www.pei.de/EN/newsroom/press -releases/year/2020/08-first-clinical-trial-sars-cov-2-germany.html;jsessionid=0C E35CB66412626071C94A446954635B.intranet212?nn=164060.

8. "Oxford COVID-19 vaccine begins human trial stage," University of Oxford, April 2020. Available at https://www.ox.ac.uk/news/2020-04-23-oxford-covid -19-vaccine-begins-human-trial-stage.

9. "Moderna Announces Positive Interim Phase 1 Data for its mRNA Vaccine (mRNA-1273) Against Novel Coronavirus," Moderna, May 2018. Available at https://investors.modernatx.com/news-releases/news-release-details/moder na-announces-positive-interim-phase-1-data-its-mrna-vaccine.

CHAPTER 8: ON OUR OWN

1. Hamilton, Isobel Asher, "Bill Gates is helping fund new factories for 7 potential coronavirus vaccines, even though it will waste billions of dollars," *Business Insider*, April 2020. Available at https://www.businessinsider.com/bill-gates -factories-7-different-vaccines-to-fight-coronavirus-2020-4.

2. Eaton, Elizabeth, "Moderna raises $500M, readies coronavirus vaccine for clin- ical testing," *Biocentury*, February 2020. Available at https://www.biocentury .com/article/304431/moderna-raises-500m-readies-coronavirus-vaccine-for -clinical-testing.

3. Jan Dams, "Donald Trump greift nach deutscher Impfstoff-Firma," *Welt*, March 2020. Available at https://www.welt.de/wirtschaft/article206555143/Corona -USA-will-Zugriff-auf-deutsche-Impfstoff-Firma.html.

4. Kelly, Éanna, "EU offers up to €80M support for German COVID-19 vaccine de- veloper reportedly pursued by Trump," Science Business, March 2020. Available at https://sciencebusiness.net/covid-19/news/eu-offers-eu80m-support-german -covid-19-vaccine-developer-reportedly-pursued-trump.

5. "Coronavirus disease 2019 (COVID-19) Situation Report—60," World Health Organization, March 2020. Available at https://www.who.int/docs/default -source/coronaviruse/situation-reports/20200320-sitrep-60-covid-19.pdf ?sfvrsn=d2bb4f1f_2.

6. "Marburg (Marburg Virus Disease)," Centers for Disease Control and Preven- tion. Available at https://www.cdc.gov/vhf/marburg/index.html.

7. "Marburg Virus Disease," World Health Organization. Available at https://www .who.int/health-topics/marburg-virus-disease/#tab=tab_1.

8. "Marburg," GSK Germany. Available at https://de.gsk.com/de-de/%C3%BCber -uns/gsk-deutschland/marburg/#geschichte.

9. Mancini, Donato Paolo, "AstraZeneca and Oxford university agree deal to de- velop virus vaccine," *Financial Times*, April 2020. Available at https://www.ft .com/content/ddf8ec8c-dc30-43b3-847e-c412704a0296.

10. "United States Securities and Exchange Commission: Form F-1 Registration

Statement," BioNTech, June 2019. Available at https://investors.biontech.de /node/7291/html.

11. Grill, Markus and Mascolo, Georg, "Biontech wollte 54,08 Euro für eine Dosis," *Süddeutsche Zeitung*, February 2021. Available at https://www.sueddeutsche.de /politik/biontech-pfizer-impfstoff-preis-eu-1.5210652.

12. "Mission Possible: The Race for a Vaccine," YouTube, April 2021. Available at https://www.youtube.com/watch?v=jbZUZ9JYNBE.

13. "COVID-19 – EU Solidarity Fund," European Commission. Available at https://ec.europa.eu/regional_policy/en/funding/solidarity-fund/covid-19.

14. "EU Vaccines Strategy," European Commission. Available at https://ec.europa .eu/info/live-work-travel-eu/coronavirus-response/public-health/eu-vaccines -strategy_en.

15. Castillo, Juan Camilo and Ahuja, Amrita et al, "Market design to acceler-ate COVID-19 vaccine supply," *Science*, March 2021. Available at https://doi. org/10.1126/science.abg0889.

16. "Shot of Hope: An Inside Look at Pfizer's Covid Vaccine," American Committee for the Weizmann Institute of Science, March 2021. Available at https://www .weizmann-usa.org/news-media/video-gallery/shot-of-hope-an-inside-look-at -pfizer-s-covid-vaccine/.

17. Balzter, Sebastian, "Eine Heldin aus Marburg," *Frankfurter Allgemeine*, April 2021. Available at https://www.faz.net/aktuell/wirtschaft/biontech-produktion -in-marburg-die-heldin-valeska-schilling-17308733.html?premium.

18. "Covid: EU's von der Leyen admits vaccine rollout failures," BBC, February 2021. Available at https://www.bbc.com/news/world-europe-56009251.

19. Crow, David and Kuchler, Hannah et al, "Trump considers fast-tracking UK Covid-19 vaccine before US election," *Financial Times*, August 2020. Available at https://www.ft.com/content/b053f55b-2a8b-436c-8154-0e93dcdb3c1a.

20. "September 7 coronavirus news," CNN, September 2020. Available at https:// edition.cnn.com/world/live-news/coronavirus-pandemic-09-07-20-intl/h_f5e 6d11e22a83184e7cce69ec0b36d3c.

21. "Coronavirus: Vaccines and Treatments," *The Washington Post*, August 2020. Available at https://www.washingtonpost.com/washington-post-live/2020/08 /07/coronavirus-vaccines-treatments/.

22. Bourla, Albert, "An Open Letter from Pfizer Chairman and CEO Albert Bourla," Pfizer. Available at https://www.pfizer.com/news/hot-topics/an_open _letter_from_pfizer_chairman_and_ceo_albert_bourla.

23. Anderson, Javonte, "America has a history of medically abusing Black peo-ple. No wonder many are wary of COVID-19 vaccines," *USA Today*, February

2021. Available at https://eu.usatoday.com/story/news/2021/02/16/black-history-covid-vaccine-fears-medical-experiments/4358844001/.

CHAPTER 9: IT WORKS!

1. Jacobs, Michael, "An Ode to Maiz from Kolkata," *Mainzer Allgemeine Zeitung*, February 2021. Available at https://www.goethe.de/ins/in/en/kultur/soc/22136897.html.

2. Pengelly, Martin, "US posts fourth consecutive daily Covid record as Joe Biden prepares taskforce," *The Guardian*, November 2020. Available at https://www.theguardian.com/us-news/2020/nov/08/joe-biden-coronavirus-taskforce.

3. Zimmer, Carl, "3 Covid-19 Trials Have Been Paused for Safety. That's a Good Thing," *New York Times*, October 2020. Available at https://www.nytimes.com/2020/10/14/health/covid-clinical-trials.html.

4. "Weekly epidemiological update," World Health Organization, November 2020. Available at https://www.who.int/publications/m/item/weekly-epidemiological-update---3-november-2020.

5. "Mission Possible: The Race for a Vaccine," YouTube, April 2021. Available at https://www.youtube.com/watch?v=jbZUZ9JYNBE.

6. "Nature's 10: ten people who helped shape science in 2020," *Nature*, December 2020. Available at https://www.nature.com/immersive/d41586-020-03435-6/index.html.

7. Thomas, Katie and Gelles, David and Zimmer, Carl, "Pfizer's Early Data Shows Vaccine Is More Than 90% Effective ," *New York Times*, November 2020. Available at https://www.nytimes.com/2020/11/09/health/covid-vaccine-pfizer.html.

8. "November-Notbremse—was gilt wo?," *tagesschau*, November 2020. Available at https://www.tagesschau.de/inland/corona-regeln-november-103.html.

9. Yen, Hope and Neergaard, Lauran and Johnson, Linda, "AP Fact Check: Trump's Claims on vaccine, election are wrong," AP News, November 2020. Available at https://apnews.com/article/election-2020-ap-fact-check-donald-trump-business-virus-outbreak-108077c4b716db604ee49b42c6d64af0.

10. Feuerherd, Ben, "Trump claims Democrats and the FDA delayed coronavirus vaccine news," *New York Post*, November 2020. Available at https://nypost.com/2020./11/10/trump-claims-democrats-and-the-fda-delayed-coronavirus-vaccine-news/

11. Chrysoloras, Nikos and Nardelli, Alberto "Astra Vaccine Haunts Countries That Shunned More Expensive Shots," Bloomberg, March 2021. Available at https://www.bloomberg.com/news/articles/2021–03–31/astrazeneca-haunts-countries-that-shunned-more-expensive-shots.

12. Gotev, Georgi and Nikolov, Krassen, "Bulgaria holds its horses with Pfizer, Moderna vaccines, puts hopes in AstraZeneca," *Euractiv*, January 2021. Available at

https://www.euractiv.com/section/health-consumers/news/bulgaria-holds-its
-horses-with-pfizer-moderna-vaccines-puts-hopes-in-astrazeneca/.

13. "Regierung gab 70 Mio. Corona-Impfdosen weg!," *Bild*, January 2021. Available at
https://www.bild.de/bild-plus/politik/inland/politik-inland/impfstoff-regierung
-gab-70-mio-corona-impfdosen-weg-74776592,view=conversionToLogin.bild
.html.

14. Adkins, William, "France denies allegations it pressured EU to buy French vaccines over German," Politico, January 2021. Available at https://www.politico.eu
/article/france-puts-down-vaccine-favouritism-allegations/.

15. "Last-minute contract closure," Peter Liese, November 2020. Available at https://www
.peter-liese.de/en/32-english/press-releases-en/3492-last-minute-contract-closure.

16. "Moderna's COVID-19 Vaccine Candidate Meets its Primary Efficacy Endpoint
in the First Interim Analysis of the Phase 3 COVE Study," Moderna, November
2020. Available at https://investors.modernatx.com/news-releases/news-release
-details/modernas-covid-19-vaccine-candidate-meets-its-primary-efficacy.

17. Steinmeier, Frank-Walter, "Nicht alle in wenigen Ländern impfen – sondern
wenige in allen Ländern," *Der Tagesspiegel*, November 2020. Available at https://
www.tagesspiegel.de/politik/bundespraesident-will-corona-impfstoff-teilen
-nicht-alle-in-wenigen-laendern-impfen-sondern-wenige-in-allen-laendern
/26634460.html.

18. Walker, Peter, "No 10 and regulator contradict Hancock's 'because of Brexit'
Covid vaccine claim," *The Guardian*, December 2020. Available at https://www
.theguardian.com/world/2020/dec/02/hancock-brexit-helped-uk-to-speedy
-approval-of-covid-vaccine.

19. "In full: 'No corners have been cut' on vaccine, says MHRA chief," YouTube,
December 2020. Available at https://www.youtube.com/watch?v=gbXo25h4ro8.

20. Reuters Staff, "EU drig watchdog urges longer approval process after UK autho-
rizes Pfizer COVID shot," Reuters, December 2020. Available at https://www
.reuters.com/article/uk-health-coronavirus-britain-ema-idUKKBN28C177.

21. Walker, Dan, "Covid vaccine: Margaret Keenan reflects receiving world's first jab,"
BBC, June 2021. Available at https://www.bbc.com/news/av/health-57532766.

22. Murray, Jessica, "Covid vaccine: UK woman becomes first in world to receive
Pfizer jab," *The Guardian*, December 2020. Available at https://www.theguardian
.com/world/2020/dec/08/coventry-woman-90-first-patient-to-receive-covid
-vaccine-in-nhs-campaign.

23. "Why two FDA members voted against the Pfizer-BioNTech vaccine,"
YouTube, December 2020. Available at https://www.youtube.com/watch?v
=2EtAzVy89ZU.

24. Peltier, Elian, "E.U.'s Top Drug Regulator Says It's 'Fully Functional' After Cyberattack," *New York Times*, December 2020. Available at https://www.nytimes .com/2020/12/10/world/europe/cyberattack-coronavirus-europe.html.

25. Engelberg, Michael, "Lights out at the EMA," *Bild*, December 2020. Available at https://www.bild.de/politik/inland/politik-inland/ema-macht-das-licht-aus-dabei -arbeiten-sie-eigentlich-rund-um-die-uhr-74497204,jsPageReloaded=true.bild.ht- ml#remId=1703072226374113611.

26. Leyen, Ursula von der, "Speech by President von der Leyen at the European Par- liament Plenary on the state of play of the EU's COVID-19 Vaccination Strat- egy," European Commission, February 2021. Available at https://ec.europa.eu /commission/presscorner/detail/en/speech_21_505.

27. Fleming, Sam, and Peel, Michael, and Chazan, Guy, "Redemption shot: von der Leyen begins fightback on EU vaccine rollout," *Financial Times*, March 2021. Available at https://www.ft.com/content/39d31c19-5a3d-4352-9bff-630f7c80e5fa.

28. Deutsch, Jillian and Herszenhorn, David, "EU countries look abroad for vaccines as doubts in Brussels grow," Politico, March 2021. Available at https://www .politico.eu/article/brussels-doubts-eu-countries-capitals-look-abroad-russia -china-coronavirus-vaccines/.

29. Reuters Staff, "EU's vaccine failure is because it didn't 'shoot for the stars,' Ma- cron says," Reuters, March 2021. Available at https://www.reuters.com/article /health-coronavirus-vaccines-macron-idCNL8N2LM6PD.

30. Kelly, Éanna, "EU's lead COVID-19 vaccines negotiator defends contracts," *Sci- ence Business*, February 2021. Available at https://sciencebusiness.net/news/eus -lead-covid-19-vaccines-negotiator-defends-contracts.

31. Martuscelli, Carlo, "Commission's Gallina pushes back on coronavirus vaccine con- tracts," Politico, February 2021. Available at https://www.politico.eu/article/sandra -gallina-european-commission-eu-coronavirus-vaccines-contracts-parliament/.

32. Krugman, Paul, "Vaccines: A Very European Disaster," *New York Times*, March 2021. Available at https://www.nytimes.com/2021/03/18/opinion/coronavirus -vaccine-europe.html.

33. "Ensuring Access to United States Government COVID-19 Vaccines," The White House, December 2020. Available at https://www.federalregister.gov/documents /2020/12/11/2020–27455/ensuring-access-to-united-states-government-covid -19-vaccines.

34. Esposito, Anthony, "'Best gift in 2020': COVID-19 vaccinations begin in Latin America," Reuters, December 2020. Available at https://www.reuters.com/article /us-health-coronavirus-mexico-vaccine-idUSKBN28Y1BT.

CHAPTER 10: THE NEW NORMAL

1. Gandel, Stephen, "Pfizer vaccine vials contain excess doses, surprising hospitals and pharmacists," CBS News, December 2020. Available at https://www.cbsnews.com/news/pfizer-covid-vaccine-vials-more-doses-expected/.

2. Kupperschmidt, Kai, "Mutant coronavirus in the United Kingdom sets off alarms, but its importance remains unclear," *Science*, December 2020. Available at https://www.sciencemag.org/news/2020/12/mutant-coronavirus-united-kingdom-sets-alarms-its-importance-remains-unclear.

3. Corum, Jonathan and Zimmer, Carl, "Inside the B.1.1.7 Coronavirus Variant," *New York Times*, January 2021. Available at https://www.nytimes.com/interactive/2021/health/coronavirus-mutations-B117-variant.html.

4. Ibid.

5. Rambaut, Andrew and Loman, Nick et al, "Preliminary genomic characterisation of an emergent SARS-CoV-2 lineage in the UK defined by a novel set of spike mutations," Virological.org, December 2020. Available at https://virological.org/t/preliminary-genomic-characterisation-of-an-emergent-sars-cov-2-lineage-in-the-uk-defined-by-a-novel-set-of-spike-mutations/563.

6. Şahin, Uğur and Muik, Alexander and Türeci, Özlem et al, "BNT162b2 vaccine induces neutralizing antibodies and poly-specific T cells in humans," *Nature*, May 2021. Available at https://www.nature.com/articles/s41586-021-03653-6.

7. Led by Christoph Prinz and Christoph Peter.

8. Klusmann, Steffen, "Ein deutsches Heldenpaar," *Der Spiegel*, December 2020. Available at https://www.spiegel.de/politik/deutschland/biontech-gruender-ugur-sahin-und-oezlem-tuereci-ein-deutsches-wunder-a-00000000-0002-0001-0000-000174691194.

9. "Vom Gastarbeiterkind zum Weltretter," *Rheinische Post*, November 2020. Available at https://rp-online.de/panorama/coronavirus/biontech-gruender-ugur-sahin-vom-gastarbeiterkind-zum-retter-der-menschheit_aid-54532197.

10. Gelles, David, "The Husband-and-Wife Team Behind the Leading Vaccine to Solve Covid-19," *New York Times*, November 2020. Available at https://www.nytimes.com/2020/11/10/business/biontech-covid-vaccine.html.

11. "Filipino nurse reflects on giving first vaccine in the UK," YouTube, January 2021. Available at https://www.youtube.com/watch?v=ugkqp0LGJtc.

12. "BioNTech alone could lift German economy by 0.5% this year – economist," Reuters, August 2021. Available at https://www.reuters.com/article/germany-economy-biontech/biontech-alone-could-lift-german-economy-by-0-5-this-year-economist-idUSL8N2PH32O.

13. Amanat, Fatima and Krammer, Florian, "SARS-CoV-2 Vaccines: Status Report," *Immunity Perspective*, April 2020. Available at https://doi.org/10.1016/j.immuni.2020.03.007.

14. "SARS: how a global epidemic was stopped," *Bulletin of the World Health Organization*, April 2007. Available at http://dx.doi.org/10.2471/BLT.07.032763.

15. "Allergic Reactions Including Anaphylaxis After Receipt of the First Dose of Pfizer-BioNTech COVID-19 Vaccine," Centers for Disease Control and Prevention, January 2021. Available at https://www.cdc.gov/mmwr/volumes/70/wr/mm7002e1.htm.

16. "A recipe for the next disaster: a new, pan-virus methodology for ramping up vaccine production," Innovative Medicines Initiative, May 2021. Available at https://www.imi.europa.eu/news-events/newsroom/recipe-next-disaster-new-pan-virus-methodology-ramping-vaccine-production.

17. "Concept paper for the development of a guideline on data requirements for vaccine platform technology master files (PTMF)," European Medicines Agency, January 2021. Available at https://www.ema.europa.eu/en/documents/scientific-guideline/draft-concept-paper-development-guideline-data-requirements-vaccine-platform-technology-master-files_en.pdf

18. Vandeputte, Joris and Saville, Melanie et al, "IABS/CEPI platform technology webinar: Is it possible to reduce the vaccine development time?," *Biologicals*, June 2021. Available at https://doi.org/10.1016/j.biologicals.2021.04.005.

19. Schlegel, Marion, "BioNTech-Chef Ugur Sahin: 'Das könnte die neue Normalität sein'," *Der Aktionaer*, February 2021. Available at https://www.deraktionaer.de/artikel/pharma-biotech/biontech-chef-ugur-sahin-das-koennte-die-neue-normalitaet-sein-20226509.html.

20. "Coronavirus: Commission signs a third contract with BioNTech-Pfizer for an additional 1.8 billion doses," European Commission, May 2021. Available at https://ec.europa.eu/commission/presscorner/detail/en/ip_21_2548.

21. Hawthorne, Jason, "Is the Market For a Flu Vaccine Disappearing?," Nasdaq, April 2021. Available at https://www.nasdaq.com/articles/is-the-market-for-a-flu-vaccine-disappearing-2021-04-04.

22. "Vaccine patent waiver could impact quality of shots -Merkel," Reuters, May 2021. Available at https://www.reuters.com/article/eu-india-merkel-idUSS8N2D400S.

APPENDIX

1. "COVID-19 Vaccines," Centers for Disease Control and Prevention. Available at https://www.cdc.gov/vaccines/covid-19/clinical-considerations/covid-19-vaccines-us.html#Appendix-C.

INDEX

Acuitas Therapeutics, 50, 113
adaptive immunity, 90
ADE. *See* antibody-dependent
    enhancement
African green monkeys, 188–89
Aimin Hui, 79, 152
Alatovic, Jasmina, 63, 123, 128, 190
ALC-0315 formulation, 51
alpha variant, 242
Altmaier, Peter, 185
animal studies, 117, 160, 162
antibodies, 74–75, 108–9, 125–26, 140
    immune system with, 19–20, 68
    monoclonal, 22, 131
    neutralizing, 66, 119, 170, 193
    spike proteins and, 68–69, 71
    T-cell response to, 127, 166–67, 233–34
    from vaccine, 121
antibody-dependent enhancement
    (ADE), 68–69, 198
antigens, 20, 22, 77, 100, 133–34
Asian flu pandemic, 13
AstraZeneca, 139, 167, 190, 206
asymptomatic cases, 64
A-U pairings, 28–29

bacteria, 95–96, 101
batch-release process, 183
Behring, Emil von, 188, 204
Bekeredjian-Ding, Isabelle, 57, 240
Bexon, Martin, 165, 198

Bhakta, Roshni, 128, 150, 152, 156, 229
Biden, Joe, 208, 211, 225
Bill & Melinda Gates Foundation, 6, 23,
    129, 220
binary coding, 25
Bingham, Kate, 193–94
BioNTech. *See specific topics*
biopharmaceutical industry, 42, 139
biosafety-level (BSL) 4 laboratories,
    118–19
BNT162b2.8 vaccine, 170–71
BNT162b2.9 vaccine, 170–71, 231–35,
    240–43
    beneficiary of, 229
    clinical trial of, 175
    data on, 200–201
    in Science Museum, 223
    stabilizing, 220
    success of, 214
    T-cell response with, 198–99
    unique achievement of, 246
Boczkowski, David, 96–97
booster shots, 241–42
Bourla, Albert, 149–50, 191, 194, 204,
    206–10
    mRNA vaccine works from, 213
    Operation Warp Speed comment of,
    227
breast cancer, 15–16
BSL. *See* biosafety-level 4 laboratories
budget, of BioNTech, 62–63

cancer
  breast, 15–16
  cells shrinking, 182–83
  coronavirus and, 38, 243–44
  drugs for, 26, 41
  from healthy cells, 18–19, 91–93
  lipids in vaccine injected for, 113
  melanoma, 33–34, 104, 182–83
  monoclonal antibodies against, 22, 131
  research on, 4–5, 18
  technologies used for, 39
  TeGenero's drug for, 55–56
  treatment of, 15, 23, 224, 234
  tumors from, 89–90
  tumor-specific antigens and, 133–34
  unique mutations in, 24
  vaccines, 90
CD4s T-cells, 117–18
CDC. *See* Centers for Disease Control
  and Prevention
cell-analysis machine, 126–27
cells, 18–19, 70, 92–93, 182–83
  DC, 90–91, 96–98, 200
  helper, 75, 117–18
  immune system using, 89–90
  protein production in, 103–4
  viruses attacking, 26–27, 101
cellular immunity, 75–76
Centers for Disease Control and
  Prevention (CDC), 15, 58, 87
CEPI. *See* Coalition for Epidemic
  Preparedness Innovations
chemical wrapper, 48–49
chicken-and-egg system, 87
childhood experience, 30–31
China, 6–9, 32, 37–38, 78–80
Cichutek, Klaus, 45–46, 57, 164, 174
clinical trials, 76–79, 161, 165–67, 172–73,
  176–78
  of BioNTech, 6, 25–26, 59, 85
  double-blind method in, 208
  for infectious diseases, 43
  lipid amounts for, 183–84
  of mRNA, 23, 43
  PEI and, 46–47, 174–75
  petitioning process for, 48

  results submitted of, 221–22
  timeline for, 134
  unexplained illnesses in, 212
  vaccines for, 39, 169–70, 180, 202–3
cloning problem, 116
Coalition for Epidemic Preparedness
  Innovations (CEPI), 129
coding segment, 101–2
cold-chain requirements, 220–21
common cold, 27, 66
contact tracing, 239
Contagion (film), 158
contagious virus, 8
control group, 225
coronavirus, 2, 6–11, 27–28, 54
  cancer benefiting from, 38, 243–44
  China's outbreak of, 32, 37–38
  crisis and reality of, 59–60
  data on spread of, 47–48
  incubation period of, 32–33
  lockdowns from, 62–63
  mutations of, 232–33
  Phase 3 trials expedited by, 208
  Poetting not worried by, 36
  positive test for, 80
  Rosenbaum company lead against, 47
  vaccines, 13–14, 26, 31, 39, 44–45,
    48–49, 163–64
cost, of vaccines, 191–93
COVID-19 vaccine, 1–2, 112–14
  of BioNTech, 151–52, 179–80, 194, 197,
    202
  manufacturing capabilities for, 181–82
  MHRA authorizing, 222
  Phase 3 trials for, 244–45
  production site for, 205–6
  unblinding study of, 212
"COVID-19 Vaccine-Maker Pledge," 207
COVID-19 virus, 63–66, 148–50, 172–74,
  201. *See also* coronavirus; SARS-
  CoV-2
  antibodies from vaccine fighting, 121
  immune response to, 166–67
Crick, Francis, 88, 93
cross-species transmission, 4
CTLs. *See* cytotoxic T-cells

CureVac (German mRNA company), 24, 45, 104, 186–87, 190
Cutter incident, 54–55
cytokine storm, 75–76, 215
cytotoxic T-cells (CTLs), 75

data, 126–27, 176–78
  on BNT162b2.9 vaccine, 200–201
  mRNA vaccines success shown in, 216–17
  novel coronavirus spread, 47–48
  from preclinical work, 35
DC. See dendritic cells
deaths, from COVID-19, 148–49
Delta variant, 241–42
dendritic cells (DC), 90–91, 96–98, 200
development process, 34–36
Diamond Princess (cruise ship), 76, 78
Diekmann, Jan, 161–62
Diken, Mustafa, 69, 99–100
DNA, 115–16, 122–23
  chemical makeup of, 28–29
  genetic code of, 93
  molecular structure of, 88
  mRNA instructions from, 93–94, 170, 203
  RNA from, 234–35
Do No Harm principle, 55
Dolsten, Mikael, 149, 201
Dormitzer, Phil, 42–43, 146, 148, 245
double-blind method, 208
Drögemüller, Johanna, 116
drugs, 41, 55, 56, 203–4

Ebola virus, 35, 118
ELISA. See immunosorbent assays
EMA. See European Medicines Agency
emergency authorization, 187–88, 208, 221
enzymes, 21, 49, 94–95, 105
Erbar, Stephanie, 109
Erich Kästner Gymnasium, 17
Ethics Commission, 166, 172–73
EU. See European Union
Europe, 11, 176, 205–6, 219

European Medicines Agency (EMA), 44, 221
European Union (EU), 195, 218–19
European VacTrain initiative, 158–59
experimental therapies, 25–26

fair pricing framework, 191
father, of Türeci, 16
Fauci, Anthony, 2, 54, 72, 103, 216–17
FDA. See Food and Drug Administration
fill-and-finish capacity, 184
first-in-human trial, 163, 170
flow cytometry machine, 102
flu vaccines, 42, 47, 148, 189
Food and Drug Administration (FDA), 44, 206, 224
Fosun company, 78–79, 148, 152–53, 156
Frieden, Thomas, 87–88

Gallina, Sandra, 226, 228
Ganymed Pharmaceuticals, 22–23, 108, 130–36, 180–81
  Phase 2 study of, 140–41
  sale of, 39
Gao, George Fu, 73
Gates, Bill, 24–25, 154, 180
gene therapy, 94, 108–9, 115, 145–46
Genentech, 139–40
genetic code, 20–22, 27–29
  of coronavirus, 7
  of DNA, 93
  of spike protein, 167–68
  of viruses, 13
Germany, 29, 190–91, 192
Ghebreyesus, Tedros Adhanom, 2, 24
globalization, 9–10, 231–32
Good Manufacturing Practice (GMP), 181
Graham, Barney, 70–72, 76, 241
grants, government, 109
Gruber, Bill, 201

Hahn, Stephen, 206
Hancock, Matt, 222
Hatchett, Richard, 239

hatred, toward Şahin, U., and Türeci, 153–54
healthy cells, 91–93
Hein, Stephanie, 77, 115–16
Heinen, Helma, 10, 100–101, 236
helper cells, 75, 117–18
Hengartner, Hans, 229
Hennig, Oliver, 183–84, 188, 205
hepatitis C, 65
Hepburn, Matt, 238–39
Hilleman, Maurice, 14
HIV. *See* human immunodeficiency virus
Huber, Christoph, 97, 99, 122, 131–32
human immunodeficiency virus (HIV), 65, 71
human trials, 41, 50–51, 55–56, 132, 163–64
humoral immunity, 74–75

immigration, 237
immune system, 14, 25–27, 89–93, 166–69
   antibodies and, 19–20, 68
   cellular and humoral immunity in, 74–76
   children's response of, 68
   cytokine storm by, 75–76, 215
   inflammation response of, 103
   internal threats recognized by, 19
   melanoma drug response of, 33–34
   mRNA response of, 23–24, 105–6, 244
   Phase 1 trial response of, 193, 213–14
   Şahin, U., understanding, 4–5
   SARS-CoV-2 response of, 214
   spike protein response of, 69–70, 217
   with T-cells, 19–20, 75–76
immunosorbent assays (ELISA), 118
immunotherapies, 17, 19, 22–23, 89
incubation period, 32–33
infectious diseases, 9–10, 23, 37, 43
   BioNTech fighting, 48
   immune system fighting, 25
   vaccines for, 110–11
influenza virus, 14–15, 58, 66, 109, 244
innate immunity, 90
innovation, 85, 108, 133–34, 192, 247

interviews, of Şahin, U., and Türeci, 217–18
intrinsic adjuvant function, 96, 111
investments, 40, 130, 132–38, 144–45
Israel, 235, 241

Jansen, Kathrin, 147, 156, 174, 200, 237
   FDA concerns and, 209–10
   quick kill strategy coined by, 197
Jeggle, Helmut, 11–12, 26, 129–32, 185, 192
Jenner, Edward, 2, 85–86, 223
Johnson, Boris, 193, 232
Johnson & Johnson vaccine, 183

kanamycin antibiotic, 116
Karikó, Katalin, 103–4, 111, 237
Kästner, Erich, 230
Katinger, Dietmar, 204
Keenan, Maggie, 1–2, 223, 238
Kent variant, 232
Kissel, Holger, 42, 144, 146–48
Kranz, Lena, 117
Kreiter, Sebastian, 34, 49, 61, 69, 94, 99
Kremer, Brad, 182
Kromayer, Matthias, 23
Krugman, Paul, 227
Kuhn, Andreas, 53, 80, 171, 179, 201, 234
Kündig, Thomas, 98

Lagkadinou, Eleni, 242
The Lancet, 7, 32
letter of intent, 151
Liese, Peter, 219
Lindemann, Claudia, 158, 161, 171, 198
lipid nanoparticles, 50–51, 183–84, 227–28, 249
   cancer vaccine injections with, 113
   formulation process of, 205
   mRNA encapsulated in, 49–50, 105–6, 116–17
lockdowns, 62–63, 187
Lockhart, Steve, 201
lymph nodes, 98, 102–3, 200
lymphoid tissue, 50

MABEL. *See* Minimal Anticipated
Biological Effect Level
Macron, Emmanuel, 226
macropinocytosis, 98
Madden, Tom, 50–53
manufacturing, 41, 181–84, 196
Marett, Sean, 36–41, 129, 139, 152, 218
business relations by, 189
Pfizer meeting with, 146–47
marriage, of Şahin, U., and Türeci,
100–101
mask wearing, 80
media coverage, 217–18
medical disciplines, 16–17, 65
meeting, of Şahin, U., and Türeci, 17–18
melanoma, 33–34, 104, 182–83
Merkel, Angela, 64, 123, 161–62, 185–86,
245
MERS. *See* Middle East respiratory
syndrome
messenger RNA. *See* mRNA
MHRA, 110, 221–22
microchips, 154
Middle East respiratory syndrome
(MERS), 8
Minimal Anticipated Biological Effect
Level (MABEL), 56
mobile manufacturing, 240–41
mobile morgues, 174
Moderna, 71–72, 139, 142, 167, 239
coronavirus collaboration of, 54
full spike approach of, 73
mRNA made by, 54
vaccine effectiveness of, 219–20
modRNA, 169–70, 177–79, 197
molecular properties, 19–20, 92–93
monoclonal antibodies, 22, 131
mortality rate, 118
Motschmann, Michael, 132, 216
mRNA (messenger RNA), 21–22, 24,
44–45, 101–4, 111–14
antigens and, 77
batch checks for, 204
BioNTech's existing platforms for, 34
cancer treatment with, 15
clinical trials of, 23, 43

COVID-19 vaccine and, 179–80, 194,
197, 202
COVID-19 virus and, 149–50
custom-made vaccines for, 182
DC injected with, 96–97
DNA instructions for, 93–94, 170, 203
drug commercialization of, 41
feasibility studies for, 180–81
genetic code needed by, 27
immune system response to, 23–24,
105–6, 244
instability of, 95
lipid-encapsulated, 49–50, 105–6,
116–17
lymph nodes injected with, 98
Moderna making, 54
as natural adjuvant, 96
Pfizer's flu vaccine with, 148
production strategy for, 53, 183–84
systemic response to, 171–72
tumor response of, 26
vaccine batch of, 116–17
vaccine unproven of, 195
mRNA vaccines, 38, 216–18, 220–21,
224–31
Bourla stating success of, 213
for influenza, 244
plug-and-play platforms for, 240–41
production of, 188
Muik, Alex, 119–22, 125–27, 201
neutralizing antibodies from, 170,
193
resourcefulness of, 176
Mukherjee, Siddhartha, 18
multiple sclerosis, 244
Munshi, Surendra, 211
mutations, 24, 232–33

Nair, Smita, 96
Narasimhan, Vas, 189
National Institutes of Health (NIH), 70
natural adjuvant, 96
Neon Therapeutics, 32, 83
NIH. *See* National Institutes of Health
Novartis, 189, 204
Nuremberg Code, 55

oncolytic viruses, 120
100 Days Mission report, 239–40
Operation Warp Speed, 36, 194, 227, 239
Oxford/AstraZeneca, 190

pandemics, 9–12, 35–37, 84, 123, 239–40
Parsons, May, 237
pathogens, 6–8, 108–9
patients, 20, 66–67, 89–90, 175
Paul Ehrlich Institute (PEI), 44–45, 166, 240
  BioNTech disagreement with, 57–58
  clinical trial notice from, 46–47, 174–75
  toxicology study rejection by, 158–59
Perlmutter, Roger, 139
Perrineau, François, 84, 123, 153
personal protective equipment, 123
person-to-person transmission, 7–8
petitioning process, 48
Pfizer, 145–55
  with BioNTech, 26, 42–43, 128–29, 202
  Operation Warp Speed inquiries to, 194
  production capacity for, 188
pharmaceuticals, 22
Phase 1 study, 35, 56–58, 159–60, 163–64
  financial markets after, 197
  immune response in, 193, 213–14
  modRNA in, 177–78
  official application for, 170
  vaccine safety in, 215
Phase 2 study, 35, 138–41
Phase 3 trials, 35, 157, 202, 208
  for COVID-19, 244–45
  efficacy and safety profiles in, 130, 224–25
plasmid, 121
plug-and-play lipids, 50
plug-and-play platforms, 240–41
pneumonia, 33, 66
Poetting, Sierk, 36, 40–41, 82–83, 153, 227, 231
  financial pitch by, 187
  start-up goals from, 62

polio vaccines, 54–55
Polymun company, 51, 212, 242
Popper, Karl, 31, 43, 60, 74, 247
preclinical studies, 34–36, 40–41, 43–44, 169
pricing framework, 191–92
Prinz, Christoph, 204, 230
procurement process, 226
production, 103–4, 171, 188, 227–31.
  See also manufacturing
  COVID-19 vaccine site for, 205–6
  facilities funded for, 144
  strategy, 53, 183–84
Project Lightspeed, 36, 39, 40–41, 77–78
  Kreiter leading, 61
  regulators and, 44
  timeline of, 161
  Vogel running, 110–11
protein production, 103–4

quick kill strategy, 197

Raine, June, 222
Ramírez, Irene, 229
receptor-binding domain (RBD), 168, 170, 193, 198
  modRNA encoding for, 179
  mutations of, 233
  of spike protein, 72–74, 114
recombinant protein subunit vaccines, 88
regulations, 44–45
respiratory diseases, 74
respiratory syncytial virus (RSV), 67
RiboMABs, 51
ribonucleic acid (RNA), 15, 20–21, 93, 234–35
Richardson, Ryan, 36–41, 78–79, 142, 184, 197
Rizzi, Ruben, 173–74, 201, 223
RNA. *See* ribonucleic acid
Röller, Lars-Hendrik, 186
Rosenbaum, Corinna, 47, 51–52, 122
Rothschild, Wilhelm Carl von, 136
RSV. *See* respiratory syncytial virus
Ryan, James, 151–52

Şahin, Ihsan (father), 30–31, 59–60
Şahin, Uğur. *See specific topics*
Sänger, Bianca, 126
saRNA. *See* self-amplifying mRNA
SARS-CoV, 9–10, 27
SARS-CoV-2, 27–29, 66–67, 232, 241–42
    ADE not issue with, 198
    BNT162b2.9 vaccine success against,
        235
    Diamond Princess with, 76
    immune response with, 214
    infections rising of, 37
    spike protein of, 72, 74, 121, 160
Schilling, Valeska, 205
school studies, of Şahin, U., and Türeci,
    16–17
Science Museum, 1–2, 223
scientific advice meeting, 45–46
scientists, 136–37
self-amplifying mRNA (saRNA), 112,
    169, 245
SEREX technology, 100
Slaoui, Moncef, 194, 209–10, 237
smallpox virus, 86
social distancing, 80, 242
Spahn, Jens, 32, 64, 187, 190
Spanish flu, 37
speech, by Şahin, U., 24–25
spike protein, 27–28, 85, 197, 233–34
    antibodies and, 68–69, 71
    full spike encoding of, 198, 200
    genetic code of, 167–68
    immune system's response to, 69–70,
        217
    RBD of, 72–74, 114
    from SARS-CoV-2, 72, 74, 121, 160
    stabilization of, 241
    VSV expressing, 121–22
staff, 41–42, 124–25
Steinman, Ralph, 90–91
Steinmeier, Frank-Walter, 220, 235–38
stock exchange, 144
Strüngmann, Andreas, 40, 132–38, 141,
    243
Strüngmann, Thomas, 40, 132–38, 141,
    216, 243

Stuart, Lynda, 23–25, 220
super-spreader events, 83–84
supply chain, 41, 233
swine flu, 14, 57–58
switchblade-like structure, 70
synthetic mRNA, 111
syringes, low dead volume, 231

taRNA. *See* trans-amplifying mRNA
task force, vaccine, 193–94
T-cells, 92, 105–6, 117–18, 198–99
    antibodies response of, 127, 166–67,
        233–34
    CTLs, 75
    immune system with, 19–20, 75–76
toxicology study, 35, 53–57, 59, 171–72
    PEI rejecting, 158–59
    results from, 221–22
trans-amplifying mRNA (taRNA), 112,
    245
translational medicine, 18, 165
Trump, Donald, 4, 55, 185, 206, 218
tumors, 100, 133–34, 140
Türeci, Özlem. *See specific topics*
two-shot regime, for vaccines, 160

uridine mRNA, 104–5, 111, 162, 168–69,
    175

vaccinations, 1–2, 42, 85–86
vaccine development, 4–5, 34–36, 177–78,
    237–38
    mRNA batch in, 116–17
    preclinical stage of, 43–44
    production process in, 171
    toxicology study in, 53–54
vaccines. *See specific topics*
venture capital firms, 132–34,
    246
vesicular stomatitis virus (VSV), 120–22,
    125–26
viral vectors, 88–89, 175
virus neutralization test (VNT),
    118
viruses, 8, 38, 120–21, 189
    cells invaded by, 26–27, 101

viruses (*continued*)
Ebola, 35
genetic sequence of, 13
influenza, 14–15, 58, 66, 109, 244
RSV, 67
SARS, 27
vaccines fighting, 33, 67–68, 86–87
zoonotic, 6–7
VNT. *See* virus neutralization test
Vogel, Annette, 109–11, 117–19, 121, 162, 170

von der Leyen, Ursula, 185, 195, 205, 226, 228
VSV. *See* vesicular stomatitis virus

wasted, vaccine percentage, 199–200
website, BioNTech not having, 109–10
Weissman, Drew, 103, 111
wet markets, 4, 7
World Health Organization (WHO), 36, 64, 123, 159

Ziegenhals, Thomas, 116
zoonotic viruses, 6–7